Joy Cometh in the Morning

Jennifer R. Vanderford

HARVEST HOUSE PUBLISHERS
Eugene, Oregon 97402

Scripture quotations in this book are from the King James Version of the Bible.

JOY COMETH IN THE MORNING

Published by Harvest House Publishers
Eugene, Oregon 97402
Library of Congress Catalog Card Number 82-083503
ISBN 0-89081-364-7

PRINTED IN THE UNITED STATES OF AMERICA.

To the Lord Jesus, my Strength, my Rock, my Refuge, my Redeemer, the Great Physician, and to David, David Jr., and Brian for their support and love.

Special thanks —

Dr. C. Everett Koop,
Surgeon General of the United States 1981

Dr. Luis Schut,
Chief of Neurosurgical Services
Children's Hospital of Philadelphia

Dr. William H. Davis, Pediatrician

Mrs. Nancy S. Davis, Mrs. Wanda Hodel, and
David Coburn, Photographers

Contents

Introduction

On Thanksgiving Day, 1980, as I sat reading my Bible in my son's hospital room, I felt impressed of the Lord to change into narrative form the diary I had been keeping:

> "That I may publish with thanksgiving, and tell of all thy wondrous works."
>
> Psalm 26:7

> "My heart is inditing a good matter . . . my tongue is the pen of a ready writer."
>
> Psalm 45:1

These two scriptures bore heavily upon my mind only hours after a doctor had told me to take my baby home and "love him until he dies."

Not only does this book tell of God's "wondrous works" but it reveals factual information that the public should know regarding their rights or the rights of their family members as patients under medical care. As a registered nurse, I knew my rights and exercised them. Sometimes a doctor's judgment and direction were not sufficient. Then, I had to rest on the verse, "If any of you lack wisdom, let him ask of God . . . " (James 1:5). Several times God's direction was not the physician's advice. God gave the wisdom for discernment, direction for His will, and the courage to follow His direction over many medical obstacles.

During my practice as a registered nurse, I was amazed at the gullibility of the general public toward medical care. "They should know their rights," I would say. Now, after my baby has had surgery four times in one year, my heart goes out to mothers who do not know their rights regarding the care of their children, and even more, to the children who are victims of careless medical procedures. I am concerned that many times patients (both young and old alike) whom the doctors assume will "never be productive anyway" seem to run an increased risk of becoming prey to experimental medical treatment or simply little treatment at all.

Sometimes doctors forget that the Lord who gave them knowledge can still direct them. They become egotistical and self-sufficient. They are offended when their actions are questioned or their advice disregarded. Psalm 94:9-10 says, "He that planted the ear, shall he not hear? he that formed the eye, shall he not see? . . . he that teacheth man knowledge, shall he not know?"

In this book, I reveal my methods of action and my determination to monitor closely the medical care that my child received. It is my prayer that this true story will give the reader the faith to put their trust in the Great Physician.

JOY COMETH IN THE MORNING

1 Feminine Intuition

It was a brisk, cool late March morning. Earlier I had gotten our sons, David Jr., age ten, and seven year old Brian, off to school. My husband David had the day off. We planned to visit my obstetrician, go shopping, have lunch together, and be home when the boys arrived from school.

As we drove through familiar streets, life in our Kernersville, North Carolina, town was going on as usual. David was quiet, concentrating on driving. But my thoughts were in turmoil. A cold fist of fear was gripping my heart.

I wanted to share my feelings with David, but I didn't want to alarm him—not until I was sure. Yet, wasn't I sure? Call it feminine intuition, whatever, I knew what I suspected was not my imagination.

We had been so excited about this baby. We enrolled in the Lamaze program and David faithfully attended classes with me. Together we planned the nursery. The walls freshly painted baby blue, decorated with beautiful plaques and pictures that would appeal to any baby. It took a lot of work to restore the old baby bed. It was the first time we had been able to decorate the nursery the way we had wanted.

We shared the baby's coming with David and Brian. They too were excited. This baby was a family goal. Our home was happy and filled with joyful anticiption.

The first finger of fear tapped me weeks before, quite by "coincidence." I know now it was the timing of the Lord. I was working as a registered nurse in ICU (Intensive Care Unit) in a large hospital. An obstetrical resident doctor came in to check on a patient in my care. After examining her he looked at me and asked, "When is your baby due?"

"April sixth."

He laughed and said, "When you get a chance I'd like to do a sonogram on you."

I knew I was unusually large for four and a half months, but I hadn't gained any weight. A few days slid by before I had the opportunity to take advantage of his offer.

Several nurses gathered around as the doctor proceeded with the sonogram. He was able to get a clear view of the baby, and a transverse measurement of its head.

"According to the baby's head measurement it should be due around March 9, instead of April 6. You must have your conception date wrong," the doctor informed me.

I stared at the baby and felt that first icy touch. Shaking my head I replied, "No, my date is accurate." Then I told him my fear.

The nurses gasped. "Jennifer! Why would you say such a thing," one scolded.

The doctor still contended that he believed I had confused my dates.

During the evening I told my family about the sonogram and that the resident doctor thought it would be early. I didn't tell them what I thought. The old saying, "Ignorance is bliss" seemed to apply in this case. So I decided to keep my suspicion to myself.

As days went by I tried to lose myself in work in order to wipe out any negative thoughts. I had recently gone through a shattering experience involving people who were thought to be my friends. Scarred from this hurt I had no desire to get close to people; consequently, I had not one with whom to share my secret feelings.

All through this pregnancy I had been unhappy and at times angry at the impersonal treatment received from the doctors and nurses who attended me. I was accustomed to routine in the medical profession, but these people were so indifferent. This group of doctors had been recommended by several nurses in the labor and delivery department of the hospital where I worked. I wanted the doctor who had attended me when Brian was born, but he was no longer delivering babies.

So I listened when the nurses assured me, "They're the best."

Just a few days earlier I had complained to one of the obstetricians during a typical visit. A nurse would hustle through checking my weight, blood pressure and urine. A doctor would take a *quick* glance at me. Sometimes he would measure my abdomen—sometimes not. The only major discomforts of my pregnancy had been chronic indigestion, pressure in the pelvic region, and during the last two weeks, episodes of projectile (forceful) vomiting. When I mentioned these problems to the doctors, they seemed to think they did not merit concern.

I began to feel like a piece of luggage on a conveyor belt. It was all so matter-of-fact. I didn't feel like a person at all, much less a pregnant lady in need of a doctor's interest and supervision.

Still pondering my growing fear, I finally became angry enough to make it known. "You all don't even know me! If I did have a problem you would've missed it with no more attention than I receive on my visits!"

Many women would not have voiced any complaints for fear their doctor might permit them to suffer more during labor in an attempt to make them regret being critical of services not rendered.

Time passed and I continued with my busy schedule. I carried my secret and shared it with no one. The obstetricians still were not concerned about my condition, and didn't even do an examination which would have alerted them that all was not well with this pregnancy.

One day in the hospital cafeteria the resident doctor who had given me the sonogram noticed I hadn't yet delivered. "You didn't have your dates mixed up, did you?"

"I told you I didn't."

"How about letting me sono you again when you have time?"

I was grateful for his concern. He seemed to be the only one. After work, a few days later, I went up to labor and delivery. He discovered on the second sonogram that the baby's head was far down into the pelvis, it was a boy and a big one. The doctor was unable to obtain a good head measurement due to the baby's position.

Again I stated my innermost fear.

He replied, "He's a big boy, probably nine or ten pounds." He paused a moment, then continued, "This machine is fairly new and I'm not as familiar with it as I should be. Why don't you let the lady in the antenatal testing lab do another one tomorrow?"

I was really getting uneasy, but didn't want to impose on the nurse's valuable time. However, a few days later I saw her in the cafeteria. After a short conversation she seemed willing to do a sonogram at my convenience.

I went to the lab during my supper hour on March 25. As she proceeded with the sonogram she confirmed the baby was a boy. His head was still lodged deep into the pelvis, and she wasn't able to get an accurate head measurement. The figure she did get was large.

Then I confided my suspicion to her. She brushed it off with, "He sure is a big boy!" She was in and out of the room several times, changing the subject when I persisted with my opinion. She did seem quite concerned when she found out I was still working a twelve-hour shift in ICU. "Why don't you go out on maternity leave?"

"Hospital policy doesn't permit a staff nurse to go on leave and retain her position in a particular unit. I really love ICU nursing. I'm only allowed three-and-a-half weeks off. This includes vacation, holiday, and accrued sick time," I explained.

"Surely they would consider making an exception," she protested.

I had worked long enough as a staffing clerk to know that policy was regarded as law and wasn't to be broken no matter who it was. Nurses were considered as numbers rather than individuals. No one was indispensable.

After a short discussion she took two photographs of the baby and said, "Take these to your doctor. Ask him to give you a due date."

Our Lamaze class was that evening. One of my doctors was to be there to answer any questions the couples might have. David had really gotten excited about being my coach during this delivery. Lamaze had not been available to us for our first two boys. Just the thought of my husband being with me during delivery made me feel more secure.

I left the lab with an aching heart, knowing all our breathing exercises wouldn't be used. A Caesarean section was inevitable even though the nurse would not confirm my self-diagnosis.

David would be so disappointed. He had become so proficient in his coaching role. He would come home from work and reprove me if I had failed to practice my breathing exercises. When should I tell him? I just couldn't bring myself to be the one to deliver the sad news.

Back in my unit I spent the last two hours of my shift attempting to lose myself again in work. The cold fist inside had tightened, and my thoughts were not cooperating with my attempts to concentrate on my job.

David and I met at Lamaze class. My question to the doctor was, "If a patient is put to sleep for a Caesarean section, can a husband still be present during delivery?"

He fumbled a little before answering "Sometimes it is permissable for the mother to be awake with an epidural for a section, and if the father wants to be present I suppose it could be arranged." It was obvious by his expression that most fathers probably wouldn't want to be present.

After class I showed the doctor my sonogram pictures. He winced, and for the first time I saw concern flicker across his face as he stared. "I can't give you a date. I'll need to talk with the nurse about this new machine before I can make a determination about these pictures."

On the drive home a contraction gripped me.

Exhausted physically and emotionally, I was just too tired to go through delivery that night. I showered, then told David and the boys about the pains, and that the sonogram revealed we were having a little boy.

"Are we still going to call him Eric?" David Jr., asked, his eyes glowing.

"We sure are," I answered, forcing a smile.

We had picked out the name Eric Heath if the baby was a boy. Sometime later we picked April for a girl.

The children finally drifted off to sleep, and my husband grew more elated as the contractions grew closer together.

We decided to go to bed, and I remember praying silently, "Lord, if I can deliver this baby without any complications, then let me give birth tonight. If there are to be complications, then allow the contractions to cease." About 11:30 p.m. they began getting farther apart, with less intensity. By midnight they had subsided completely. I felt the baby change position, and I too drifted into much needed sleep.

The next morning I pondered my request to the Lord and His answer. There would be complications if the doctor allowed me to attempt a vaginal delivery.

As we drew near the doctor's office I wanted to cry. But I knew if I let go, the secret I had worked so hard to keep would come blundering out. I still wanted to protect David as long as I could. Inside I felt like jelly. In the next few minutes they would tell me something definite that would confirm my deepest fears. It would be a relief to hear it from the doctor. Yet I dreaded it. David would have to know. I hoped he would be told tactfully. I still didn't want to be the one to bring such sad news.

The baby moved and I was strangely comforted by his active kicking. One thing I knew for sure. Our unborn son was very much alive.

David eased the car to a stop, and we entered the building.

Our lives would never be the same again.

2

Bad News

Upon arriving at the doctors' office, we were both escorted without delay to the sonogram room. I hadn't counted on David accompanying me there. My hands grew cold and clammy. Today I was treated more like a person than a piece of luggage.

Although the room was small, I was receiving the undivided attention of two nurses and two doctors; and of course David stood quietly. Oh! How I wished I had prepared him more for what was about to happen. I was angry at myself for not being more open with him.

I finally positioned myself up on the examining table. I looked like a blimp standing on end. The gel on the scanner was cold. I began to shiver uncontrollably. "Do you want to see the baby's parts?" the doctor asked as he pressed the scanner firmly on my abdomen.

I was angry with myself for allowing this to happen to David. Closing my eyes and turning my head in the opposite direction, I cooly answered, "I've already seen them several times."

I didn't want to look at David. I wanted to block out this whole experience. I couldn't bear the hurt in his eyes if he figured out what was wrong.

To my surprise the doctor very bluntly began to voice his diagnosis. "She's hydromnios," (meaning there was a lot of accumulated fluid in my abdomen.) He continued, "Yes, the baby's hydrocephalic. Look at the enlarged ventricles. I doubt if it will live; and if it does, it will be grossly abnormal.

I was right. I was carrying a waterhead baby. I opened my eyes and looked at David. The doctor had not only "spilled the beans," he had said two things that I was not ready for: "I doubt if it will live; and if it does, it will be grossly abnormal." The words rang bitterly in my mind.

David was holding together well. For his sake I tried also. I was furious with the doctor for being so candid. Surely, he could have thought of a more tactful way of telling us his diagnosis.

Everyone except David left while I got dressed. Then we sat down, speechless, holding hands while waiting for the doctor to return. I felt so guilty; I wished David would fuss at me for not telling him. I was fighting back tears. Why was I so intent on protecting him? He has always been very strong and capable of handling me at my lowest point.

The door opened, interrupting the deadly silence. It was the other doctor who was with us during the sonogram. His manner was much more tactful and gentle. He said, "The baby is breech, no longer down into the pelvis. Due to the baby's head size and his position, a C-section is in order."

When a mother attempts to deliver a hydrocephalic baby, she and the baby face danger. If the baby's head should become lodged in the birth canal, it would necessitate decompression. (This is achieved by inserting a needle to draw off fluid from the brain to decrease the baby's head size, facilitating delivery; this usually kills the baby instantly.)

He mentioned the doctor's name that had just completed the sonogram. (I'll refer to him as Doctor Smith.) My eyes began to fill with tears as I held tightly to David's hand. "Doctor Smith will actually do the section, and I will assist Saturday morning at eight o'clock if that's okay with you both." We nodded. He lowered his voice and continued, "Doctor Smith only gives this baby a ten to twenty percent chance of living. The head is very large, and many times these babies just won't breathe well on their own."

A big tear fell down my cheek. I knew that if a large amount of fluid had accumulated in the baby's head, it would depress the respiratory center in his brain and would account for his inability to breathe. The doctor went on, "We'll give you an epidural and also put you to sleep."

We nodded understandingly. Tears were flowing

freely now. I said, "Well, if he can't lead a normal life, then it will be gracious if the Lord sees fit to take him on to heaven at birth."

The doctor nodded and told us the receptionist was making arrangements for my admission to the hospital at three o'clock the following afternoon.

We left the office and sat in the car for a while to collect and share our thoughts. The Lord gave us both strength and composed our emotions, allowing us to get things into perspective.

Since I was having a Caesarean section, even without complications, I would be hospitalized for at least five days. This would prevent me from sharing the burden of arranging the details and attending the funeral of our little boy.

I didn't want the entire burden to rest on David's shoulders. After a brief discussion, we agreed we should go by the funeral home, pick out a casket, and make tentative arrangements.

I was scheduled to work on Friday. We stopped by the hospital to let my head nurse know of our circumstances. While we talked with her, I insisted that she permit me to come to work the next day and allow me to work up until my admission time.

She was reluctant. I argued that it would keep my mind occupied and would help me to overcome the depression that I was sure would overwhelm me if I stayed at home. After further consideration and the "okay" from our supervisor, she consented.

After leaving the hospital, David and I went by the funeral home as we had planned. We explained our predicament to the funeral director who greeted us and asked if we would pick out a casket.

He was very helpful and understanding. We chose a moderately priced casket and vault and left our name with him. Several years before we had purchased some cemetery property, and we discussed the plot we would use.

When we finished, David took me to lunch. Even though our appetites were completely gone, we knew we needed to eat something. We stopped by one of our favorite restaurants and tried to choke down some of the food.

The lump in my throat seemed to swell, and I wasn't very successful with my attempt to eat. David did better, but I could tell he was trying to put up a good front for me.

We left the restaurant and decided to go by my mother's house and deliver the news in person. My father had died fourteen years before, and my mother's health was failing. We dreaded her physical and emotional reaction. Excluding David and myself, I didn't know of anyone else more excited about this baby's arrival.

Reluctantly, we knocked at her door. Sitting down together in her living room, we told her as gently as we could what the doctors had said. The Lord sustained her in a sweet way.

Tearfully, we all prayed together. We asked the Lord to take the baby at birth and prevent him from suffering if he were not able to lead a normal life. I thought silently that I could cope with the baby's homegoing at birth easier than I could adjust to a "grossly abnormal" baby. I prayed, "Nevertheless, not my will, Lord, but Thine be done."

A short time later, we left and picked up the boys at school. Of all days, David Jr. had gotten the maximum amount of demerits for talking in class. Several weeks earlier I had warned him that if his demerits ever totaled thirty, he would get a spanking from me in addition to any punishment his teacher chose to give him.

He had always been honest with me about any reproof he received for misbehavior. As he walked to the car with a long, sad face, I knew something was wrong. When I questioned him he confessed the reason for it. Since I had promised the disciplinary action, I felt obligated to follow through, even though David offered to take care of it.

After I disciplined David Jr., I held him on what little lap I had and told him how much I loved him and why I wanted him to be obedient and learn to practice self-control. It had always been my custom to cuddle and love my boys after any punishment I had to give.

After he gained composure, we both went into the den where Brian and David were sitting quietly. Once again, David and I went through the same news with the boys. We prayed with them. I was surprised they took it so hard. For some reason, I thought their ages would allow them to accept the news in a more detached manner than they did.

They had numerous questions. We answered them honestly and to the best of our ability, but the answers didn't seem to satisfy the "why." Since we could not understand "why," we weren't able to answer that one big dominant question for them.

After we talked with them at length, I decided I must put forth my best effort to keep their routine as normal as possible. Supper had to be prepared, and groceries purchased so they would have enough to eat during my hospital stay. I encouraged them to do their homework while I slipped quietly into the nursery.

I quietly picked up my packed suitcase and carefully removed all the baby clothes. I laid on the baby's chest-of-drawers the outfit in which I wanted him to be buried. I wanted to make everything as easy for David as possible.

I wanted to take the baby's bed down and pack away everything that pertained to a baby. I knew of no one of our intensive care patients who had lived when the doctors only gave a ten to twenty percent chance of survival. I didn't think I could bear disassembling the nursery after returning home empty-handed.

Something kept me from taking everything down. I was really too emotionally and physically exhausted to tackle such a chore. Besides, it was past supper time; and I simply had to go to the grocery store.

After my grocery shopping, I tore into my household chores as any expectant mother would if she knew her exact time of hospitalization. The wash had to be caught up and the house made neat and in order before I left for work in the morning.

When I finally went to bed, I was past exhaustion. I thought surely, as tired as I was, I would fall asleep immediately. Instead, I lay awake while Eric kicked inside me.

I felt guilty permitting a C-section, knowing Eric's removal from his safe environment would take his life. For a few seconds, I wanted to die during childbirth. If Eric couldn't live, then I did not want to either.

My common sense told me a section must be done, but I enjoyed feeling Eric kick. Many times I had accused him of playing football. It would suit me fine if I never woke up to the emptiness I would have to face without this little one I had already learned to love.

The Lord rebuked me, reminding me of the two precious boys I already had and the husband with which He had blessed me. I said, "I know Lord, but the depression that will overwhelm me after this loss, will surely render me an inadequate wife and mother." He seemed to rebuke me a second time and challenged me trust Him.

I glanced at the clock. It was after midnight. David had been in the bed for at least an hour. "Was he asleep?" I wondered. "David?" I asked softly, testing to see if he still happened to be awake.

"Yes," he answered clearly.

"You weren't asleep?"

"No."

"Do you still want to be with me during my section?"

"Do you think they'll let me?"

"They will, if we insist. Do you want to be there?"

"I'd like to, if you want me to."

"Then we'll tell the doctor you want to be there. Since I'm having an epidural, there's no reason I should be asleep. So I'll tell him that I want to be awake. This way we'll both be able to see the baby alive together. He will probably live at least a few minutes after birth. We'll still share this experience together as we had planned, okay?"

"Okay."

"Well, goodnight."

"Goodnight."

I had wondered why he hadn't talked about his being able to observe, as we had planned, through Lamaze classes. Then it dawned on me. He was trying to let me bring up the subject. He knew I was a barrel full of tears and wasn't about to cause a break in it by bringing up the subject.

No one could have been more understanding and protective than the sweet guy I was lying beside. I loved him so! I felt I was such a failure to him and my two precious boys asleep in the next room. I wouldn't be bringing home the baby I had promised and built up the excitement for during the past nine months. It must have been about one o'clock a.m. when I finally drifed off to sleep.

3
Coping

I was up at five a.m. getting ready for work. I tried hard to cover my swollen eyes with make-up. I knew my head nurse had briefed everyone to avoid the subject of my pregnancy; still, I was afraid I would burst into tears if anyone even glanced at me wrong.

I took my suitcase to work so that I could leave the floor and go straight to Admitting. I became totally engrossed with the care of my patients. I decided that since I had made plans for Eric's death, I should also make plans for his survival.

The normal procedure for hydrocephalic newborns was to feed them in our own special-care nursery for their first forty-eight hours. If they survived these two days, they were then sent to a nearby hospital for a shunt (a tube passed from the enlarged ventricles down to the abdomen, allowing the excess fluid to drain from the brain to the peritoneal region; consequently, being filtered through the kidneys to the bladder and out through the urine).

If the shunting procedure were to be successful, then the baby's fontanels would be allowed to close; thus, the results could be a perfectly normal looking baby within three or four months.

I decided I didn't want my baby to go to any other hospital. As far as I was concerned, no one could top our very own neurosurgeons. When my preferred neurosurgeon came to our unit that morning, I followed him into the nurses' station and asked if he still treated hydrocephalic infants. He assured me that he did and graciously consented to assess and treat mine if he survived.

On my morning break, I called our children's pediatrician and told him of my scheduled section and what the obstetricians had predicted. I emphatically told him of my decision to leave Eric at this hospital and of the neurosurgeon who was to treat him if he should survive. He assured me that my wishes would be honored.

I knew many of the staff nurses and by now the news of my unfortunate situation had made its way around the hospital. I knew many would be genuinely interested, while others would be just curious.

At lunch, in the hospital cafeteria, I was able to talk with our director of nurses. I emphasized that while the baby lived, I did not intend for him to be a side-show in our special care nursery. I asked that she relay the message to the nurse in charge not to permit other hospital personnel to see him without my permission. After all, it was unusual for our nursery to keep "grossly abnormal" babies. She was very understanding and assured me that my instructions would be carried out.

For the rest of the afternoon, I kept myself busy with my patients.

The tears welled up only twice as I made my way to the linen cart. I asked the Lord to give added grace and strength, and He did just that. For the first time in my life, I was realizing what the Bible meant in II Corinthians 12:9 " . . . my strength is made perfect in weakness . . . ." I had never been weaker physically or emotionally in my life, but it was such a comfort to know that the Lord was with me. I felt His strength carrying me through. His presence was so real and so sweet.

At three o'clock I left the unit and went to Admitting. It was four-thirty before I was finally escorted to my room. The hour and a half seemed to drag by. It was impossible to keep my mind occupied. I caught myself dwelling on the situation that I had tried so desperately to avoid. It was raining outside, adding to my gloom.

I began to blame myself for working during my entire pregnancy. I never could go at a moderate pace. I loved nursing. I had tried to look after my patients as if they were my family members. I would get so engrossed in my work that I didn't remember to take a break and would work past the hour when my shift changed.

The nursing shortage was beginning to manifest itself in our unit, especially on the evening shifts. I tried to do all the little extra things that I knew the next shift would not have time for. I had been able to obtain a permanent day shift position (which wasn't the easiest thing to accomplish). It was the only shift I could work and still be an adequate wife and mother.

Our hospital policy would not permit a staff nurse to go on a maternity or medical leave of absence for even six weeks and return to her same position. I only had four-and-a-half weeks of time built up that I could take without going on leave. Thus, I chose to work until time for delivery, returning in four-and-a-half weeks in order to keep my position.

We had twelve-hour shifts, and many days I could hardly walk to the car after work because of exhaustion and enormous pressure in the pelvic region. Did I cause this baby added distress and problems? I was so determined to hang on to something I loved. Was it worth the cost? Would I even be able to return to work in four-and-a-half weeks? Would my determination be fruitless? Suddenly, I felt myself growing bitter toward hospital policies.

I recalled occasions when X-ray technicians would come into the unit to do portable chest X-rays on our patients. I tried to be very careful to protect myself. Several times I would be caring for a patient on the other side of a curtain from where the technicians would be preparing to make an

X-ray. I would caution them to let me know before they actually took the X-rays, so I could leave the room. Instead, they forgot and would make the X-ray without warning me. Did this cause Eric's condition?

Maybe I should have quit work as soon as I knew I was pregnant; no career was worth a baby's life or health. I had told my obstetricians of the X-ray incidences. They had assured me it was nothing to be concerned about. I felt the baby kick, and again the feeling that tomorrow he may never kick again gave me a horrible feeling.

By the time I reached my room, David had arrived from work. He went out to get us some sandwiches. Again, I tried to choke down food. After all, it would be my last good meal for a while, and at the same time David would feel better if I ate.

I managed to eat the sandwich, although it felt like lead in my stomach. David watched television; I wondered if he were really interested in the programs. I pretended to watch with him, but my mind was only on the baby.

We waited for three hours for a doctor or nurse to come in and talk with us—yet no one had come. None of the usual routine of admitting a patient had been carried out. I found myself wishing I had worked my complete twelve-hour shift. Why was it so important that I be admitted at three o'clock, when it was obvious no one on the floor had time for me.

David said, "I wish the doctor would come by, so we can tell him I want to be with you, and that you want to be awake for the baby's delivery."

"I know; so do I," I answered. I knew by his statement that he wasn't as engrossed in the television as he had seemed.

Around seven-thirty I heard nurses rolling babies from the nursery to their mothers for feeding. The babies were whimpering and crying. Of all the heartaches of the past two days, this had to be the most unbearable moment. I knew David heard them, but he fixed his eyes on the television.

I turned my head away from him. I thought I had already cried my tear ducts dry the night before, but again my eyes filled with tears, trickled down my face, and fell on the white uniform I was still wearing. How horrible it would be tomorrow to hear those same sounds and know that I would never get to have Eric brought to me. Again—selfishly—only for a moment—I wanted to die on the delivery table. I went to the bathroom to dry my eyes and compose myself.

Just then, one of the anesthesiologists came in. We were able to convey our wishes to him regarding David's presence and my remaining awake during delivery. He seemed very understanding and cooperative.

Shortly after he left, a resident doctor came in apparently just to chat. He told me during the conversation that I should be thankful I found the condition of the baby on the sonogram. He stated, "In the past, when mothers have attempted to deliver hydrocephalic babies by normal delivery—in cases where the baby's head was too large to pass through the birth—a large needle would be inserted into the baby's head, drawing off the fluid to facilitate delivery. This rapid decompression is immediately fatal to the baby." He asked a few questions and left.

My thoughts began to rampage. What if I hadn't taken my sonogram picture to my doctors? How horrible it would've been to have endured a long, difficult, fruitless labor causing added distress to the baby, only to have its life ended so abruptly! Could I have endured such a labor as exhausted as I was physically? The Lord had directed miraculously in spite of my doctors.

Minutes later, Doris, a dear nursing friend from labor and delivery recovery room, came in. It was her duty to inform me and to prepare me for the sensations I would encounter during my epidural, and also what to expect from the epidural effects. She did a good job, and then said, "I'm off tomorrow; but if you don't mind, I'd like to come back and be close by to show David around and help him. Just in case he needs to leave the delivery room, I could be there."

I said, "That would be nice, but I don't want you to feel you have to come back on your day off."

"I want to, if that's okay with David," she replied.

"Sure, that would be fine," he agreed.

Only the Lord knows how much Doris meant to me at that moment. Not only did I want her there to be with David, I wanted her there to supervise the doctors! I had lost all respect for their ability and judgment for office visits, much less for their surgical expertise!

To top it all off, *not one of the five doctors had even*

poked his head in my door that afternoon or evening. Finally, one of the staff nurses came in and hurried through the routine of admitting me.

My neighbor Frances was the only person outside of my family that I had told about Eric and my scheduled section. She also was sent from heaven! She came in with a lovely bowl of flowers. How she managed to get in, I do not know. The hospital rules were bent, I think, since only immediate family is allowed in the obstetric units.

Only moments earlier, as I had heard the babies cry, I reached my lowest ebb. Thinking to myself it was too much to bear, the Lord lifted the burden by sending two of the sweetest friends any one could be privileged to have. Frances stayed only a short time; but she shared with me her experience of losing triplets, then the trials of two beautiful baby girls born with cleft palates. After she left, I felt I could face whatever was ahead for me.

David and I finally decided the doctors weren't coming, so he left the hospital around ten-fifteen p.m. I proceeded to shower and get into bed.

Total exhaustion claimed me.

4

Soul-Searching

Around two-thirty a.m. I awoke. My mind swept back through the years.

I had been brought up a preacher's kid. My dad, a very conservative fundamentalist, preached the punishment of God when one of His children sins. As a consequence, anytime things went wrong in my life, whether physical or financial, I was accustomed to wonder immediately for what sin I was being chastised. Life's difficulties were not always chastisement for a Christian, I knew; however, I would always begin soul-searching when things went wrong. This time was no exception.

The past year and a half had been very difficult for me in my own Christian life. I had gone through a very disappointing experience with so-called "good Christian friends." It had left me spiritually limp; and only by God's grace was my life not totally shipwrecked.

My work as a nurse had been healthy for me both emotionally and spiritually. Nevertheless, I hesitated to make friends or trust anyone. I decided keeping my distance from friendship was the safest way not to be hurt. I felt let down—that no one understood me except my family and the Lord. I was especially skeptical of "church members."

While working as a nurse, I had observed people who didn't even profess Christianity treating others with more kindness and concern than the circle of people with whom I had recently been associated. You know the type: pious, sanctimonious, critical, envious gossips. Those are the kind who spend so much time scrutinizing the lives of others that they forget the simplest manifestation of discipleship: "By this shall all men know that ye are my disciples, if ye have love one to another" (John 13:35). When you don't measure up to their standards, then you're avoided and put down. Just when you're at your lowest point, they forget Galatians 6:1—"Brethren if a man be overtaken in a fault, ye which are spiritual, restore such an one in meekness; considering thyself, lest thou also be tempted."

They pretend to be "concerned" when they decide others should know your problems (their version of your problems) so everyone can "pray" for you. Instead of extending an effort to restore you, they wouldn't throw a rope if you were drowning! Toward the end of my second trimester of pregnancy, the Lord provided "a way of escape" from that type of people.

My husband made a long overdue decision to change our church membership. I cautioned him not to ever again expect me to be involved in church activities to the extent I had been in the past.

I was perfectly content to teach my kids the Bible in our home, except for the fact that I knew that the Bible teaches "Not forsaking the assembling of ourselves together . . . " (Hebrews 10:25). Therefore, I promised him I would be faithful to church attendance, and nothing else! Furthermore, I had no desire to make friends or to get involved. He said lovingly that he understood, but that he felt we should still make the change.

Not long after joining another church, we had a visiting soloist. He gave his testimony. While he spoke, he told of a trial in his life. One of his children, a little girl, was born mentally and physically retarded. He told how this trial had given his life new direction.

Ironically, his little girl had been born on the very day that my baby was due. He and his wife had named her *the exact first and middle name* that I had picked out if my baby should be a girl. I shuddered inside and cried as he talked. This incident occurred shortly after the first sonogram that had left me strongly suspicious of Eric's hydrocephalus condition. I had difficulty concentrating on the rest of the service. Was the Lord trying to prepare me for something similar? I wondered.

That night after church, I had trouble falling asleep. I prayed a silent prayer, something like this:

> "Now Lord, you know I'm not very strong spiritually anymore. I'm trying hard to get on my feet from my last spiritual set-back. I couldn't handle an abnormal baby. A trial like this would be more than I could bear at this time. It wouldn't make me a better Christian. It would ruin me for good. I'd get bitter, Lord. Besides, all my ex-friends would be sure that I had committed some terrible sin if something like that came my way. They always thought that when others had trials. Surely, you wouldn't permit this to happen to me. Now Lord, if our baby is hydrocephalic, you just make it well before delivery. Okay?
> Goodnight, Dear Lord."

I felt like my prayer didn't go any higher than the ceiling. Then I turned quietly to David and said, "Honey, are you awake?"

"Yes."

"I've decided not to name our baby April if it's a girl. I'm going to pick out another name."

"Okay," he said sleepily.

****

It was after three a.m., and my past continued to drift through my mind like a diary. I had been involved "up to my neck" in church service from my childhood, but many times I had not stayed close to the Lord. Being involved in a church doesn't mean a person is a Christian.

The Bible says in Roman 3:23, "For all have sinned, and come short of the glory of God," I knew that included me, and it seemed I was remembering all my failures and mistakes. I realized how short I had fallen and how often I had sinned! Was this experience chastisement? I came to the conclusion that if it were, then I did not deserve the two healthly children I had, nor any of God's blessings. I realized what a contrite spirit was for the first time in my life.

I began to pray, confessing every wrong doing that had crossed my mind. Many sins I had confessed and forsaken years before, yet I asked the Lord's forgiveness again. Some more recent faults and failures He brought to my remembrance.

Bitterness had crept its way into my life, and I knew I must forsake it to have real victory and peace. The urge to pick up my Bible and open it strongly overwhelmed me. Opening to Psalms 34:18 I read, "The Lord is nigh unto them that are of a broken heart; and saveth such as be of a contrite spirit."

As I continued to read at random (later I realized the Lord was bringing to my attention the exact passages I needed) I felt the Lord's presence so sweetly.

> "Have mercy upon me, O Lord, for I am in trouble, mine eye is consumed with grief . . . "
>
> Psalm 31:9
>
> "I sought the Lord, and he heard me, and delivered me from all my fears."
>
> Psalm 34:4

> "Be of good courage, and he shall strengthen your heart, all ye that hope in the Lord."
>
> Psalm 31:24
>
> "Let me not be ashamed, O Lord; for I have called upon thee . . . "
>
> Psalm 31:17
>
> "For his anger endureth but a moment; in his favor is life: weeping may endure for a night, but joy cometh in the morning."
>
> Psalm 30:5

Then He reminded me of the scripture in the New Testament that referred to the blind man Jesus healed: "And as Jesus passed by, he saw a man which was blind from his birth. And his disciples asked him, saying, Master, who did sin, this man, or his parents, that he was born blind? Jesus answered, Neither hath this man sinned, nor his parents: but that the works of God should be made manifest in him" John 9:1-3.

With this thought, I had peace that even though I deserved chastisement, this experience wasn't being sent to me as punishment. I continued to read the Psalms in a more orderly fashion. They were just what I needed, so richly comforting and sweet.

I became engrossed with my Bible. I wondered why I had neglected it. For some reason my mind kept returning back to Psalm 30:5—" . . . weeping may endure for a night, but *joy cometh in the morning*." (Italics added)

Weeping had definitely endured for two nights now; but how, Lord, will I possibly have joy in the morning? How can I have joy if my baby dies? Then He brought another blessed verse to my attention. Psalm 6:5—"For in death there is no remembrance of thee: in the grave who shall give thee thanks?"

My heart leaped with joy! Now I had peace that something wonderful was truly going to happen! I began to wonder how the Lord was going to let my baby live. Death would not bring me "joy in the morning." "Grossly abnormal" would not bring me "joy in the morning." Could it be that the Lord would make Eric perfect before the doctors took him from my womb? I couldn't comprehend just how, but I knew that "joy in the morning" was coming to me! God had promised me, and I knew nothing was impossible with him!

I had probably slept only six hours out of a total of forty-three, but I was much too excited now to sleep. With great anticipation, I looked forward without dread or fear to morning!

It was around four-thirty a.m. when a nurses' aid came into my room to prepare me for surgery. The calm peace and assurance lingered. I felt the presence of the Lord in my life as never before, surpassing the times when I was so actively serving at church. His presence was so sustaining. It seemed as though He were holding me right in the palm of His strong hand.

The aid worked rapidly, complaining she was behind in her work. I knew what she needed to do and began to help her. My abdomen had to be shaved and washed with an antiseptic soap solution. The solution is prepackaged in a prep kit.

Since it is supposed to be sterile, warm water cannot be added from the faucet.

I knew that for all abdominal surgeries, the patient had to be catherized (a tube slipped into the bladder, allowing urine to drain into a bag, preventing the bladder from becoming full during surgery). I wanted to make sure she did it right, but I definitely could not see to supervise or assist. As rushed as she was, I anticipated she would hurry through this procedure carelessly. Sure enough, I was right! Her technique on catherization left a lot to be desired. I began to have bladder spasms; but even with that discomfort, I still had peace and contentment within.

David arrived around seven-thirty a.m. and watched as I was transferred from my bed to the labor and delivery stretcher. My friend Doris arrived and began "to show David the ropes" attempting to make him more comfortable in his strange environment.

They rolled me into a room where the anesthesiologist began preparing me for my epidural. Very calmly and explicitly, as he worked, he told me what to expect moment by moment during the epidural induction. He also told me to let him know if I felt a considerable amount of discomfort at any time.

I was still shivering from the preparation back in my room, and probably from nervous excitement. I tried with difficulty to hold still as he inserted the needle into my back. He managed to get it in okay in spite of my body's lack of cooperation! One of the side effects of the epidural is shivering! Consequently, I felt my body quivering uncontrollably. The nurse brought extra blankets, but nothing seemed to help.

Shortly, Doris brought David into the room. He was completely dressed in scrub clothes. He looked so cute! He would've made a nice looking doctor himself, I thought. His presence next to me was comforting. My shivering even began to subside. Everything seemed to be going just fine until my doctor arrived.

He looked at David. "Is he going to be here?" he asked with a grimace on his face.

After a moment of silence I replied, "We talked it over, Doctor, and decided we wanted to do it this way. I had planned to tell you, but you never came by after my admission yesterday."

"Well, you're going to be asleep," he said in an ordering way.

I continued, "No, we both want to see this baby alive together."

He huffed, "You're just going to make it hard on me and you!" He turned abruptly toward the door.

"Dr. Smith," I continued, "don't worry about me; just make a large enough incision to get the baby out with the least distress to him."

He stopped. "Then you don't mind a mid-line incision?" he asked.

"No, I don't show my belly in the summertime anyway."

"Well, that will make it a little easier," he gruffed as he left the room.

The anesthesiologist talked to me reassuredly. "If at any time you feel you need to go to sleep, we can arrange it. If the pressure you feel during the procedure becomes unbearable, we can also knock the edge off by allowing you to breathe a little nitrous oxide. Just let me know what your wishes are. We'll be able to communicate with each other throughout the entire operation as long as you wish to remain awake."

"I understand." I wondered why more doctors and nurses didn't have the bedside manner of an anesthesiologist! The Lord used him to keep me calm when my confidence might have been destroyed to the point that I would have followed the doctor's orders instead of my wishes, and better judgment.

5

Tears of Joy

My epidural didn't take effect as fast as the anesthesiologist desired. Around 8:10 a.m. I was transferred to the labor and delivery operating room. I could still feel the anesthesiologist touch my thighs when I should have been numb up to my waist—the one I used to have!

Dr. Smith came in, scrubbed and ready. The anesthesiologist asked him to wait five more minutes. "She's not quite ready yet." Dr. Smith grunted that he had another delivery to go to and began to proceed with my section anyway.

It was quite uncomfortable as he began clipping the outer layer of skin. I thought to myself that he probably wanted me to beg to be put to sleep. It made me even more determined I wasn't going to sleep, especially now!

The Lord's grace was sufficient; and the anesthesiologist must have rushed the epidural medication, because shortly I only felt pressure, not pain. I clinched David's hand as twenty minutes seemed like an hour. The anesthesiologist and I talked throughout the operation.

At eight-thirty a.m. our precious little boy was delivered. He was handed to the nurse, and she carefully laid him in the crib next to me. He looked normal except for his head size. He was very cyanotic (blue in color) and not very active. I watched intensely, anxious for him to breathe and turn pink.

I reached out and softly stroked his dark hair. "Eric, honey, Mommy loves you. I'm sorry if I did something to cause this, Sweetheart." My voice began to quiver as I spoke. My faith weakened because his color was poor and was not improving as fast as it should. I continued to stroke him gently and then asked, "He's not going to make it, is he?" No answer. The nurse was careful not to even show expression. "I'll see you in heaven. Mommy and Daddy love you."

Seconds later, he began to turn pink, and my faith grew stronger. "I think he's going to make it after all. May I hold him?"

The nurse said "no." My fingerprints and his footprints were made. I continued to stroke him, and he began to wiggle like he should. His eyes were opening some, and I repeated, "I sure would love to hold him."

The anesthesiologist said, "Wrap that baby up, and give him to his mother!" Thank the Lord for anesthesiologists! My arms were weak and shaky from the epidural. My husband helped stabilize him in my left arm and hovered near talking to Eric softly and sweetly.

He began to whimper and wiggle his nine-pound four-and-a-half ounce form. His head was not as large as I had anticipated, and to me he was beautiful! He became even more adorable as his color continued to improve and his dark eyes squinted open under the bright room light.

Sweet peace swept over me; for at this very moment, I knew he was going to live. My weak, shaky voice broke periodically as I looked at him through my tear-filled eyes and sang:

Far away in the depths of my spirit
(today)
Rolls a melody sweeter than psalm;
In celestial-like strains it unceasingly falls
O'er my soul like an infinite calm.
Peace! peace! wonderful peace,
Coming down from the Father above;
Sweep over my spirit forever, I pray,
In fathomless billows of love.

—Cooper

The doctors sutured my incision as I continued to sing and hold the sweetest baby in the whole world:

Jesus loves (you) this I know,
For the Bible tells (us) so;
Little ones to him belong,
(You) are weak, but *He* is strong.

Yes, Jesus loves (you),
Yes, Jesus loves (you),
Yes, Jesus loves (you),
The Bible tells (us) so."

—Bradbury

I cuddled Eric closely as he tilted his head toward me. The whimpering stopped, his eyes closed in sweet contentment. Then he slept quietly nestled between his daddy and mommy. Such a cherished moment I shall never forget! How glad I was now that I had insisted on staying awake!

A nurse entered and said that the pediatrician was there to see him. Reluctantly, we let our little one leave with her. The obstetricians finished, and *without a word*, left. I was wheeled into the recovery room with David at my side. The anesthesiologist came into give me another dose of the epidural medication to permit longer relief of pain before removing the IV needle from my back. We were in the recovery room only a short while before Eric's pediatrician came in to talk with us.

"Jennifer, I can't find a thing wrong with the baby except the size of his head. His Dubowitz test (neurological assessment on the newborn) score was good. I'm going to call Dr. Johnson (fictional name of Eric's neurosurgeon) and let him look him over."

I wasn't surprised at his findings but was elated to the point of tears. I already knew Eric was going to be okay, but every new piece of information seemed to confirm it. Therefore, I waited with anxious anticipation to hear the news that should come from my neurosurgeon.

I was back in my room when he arrived. He confirmed that Eric manifested no neurological deficiencies and stated he expected a brain scan to show what is termed Dandy-Walker hydrocephalus.

"This is the best type to have, and usually the easiest to correct," he said. "In this type of hydrocephalus, the fourth ventricle of the brain is obstructed—causing the cerebral spinal fluid to accumulate, forming a huge cyst. This is corrected by shunting the cyst (a tube inserted into the enlarged ventricle—running just under the skin of the abdomen—where the excess fluid is drained into the abdominal cavity and is absorbed by the kidneys and excreted with the urine). Many of these babies grow normally and lead normal lives. We'll know more when his brain scan is done on Monday," he concluded.

That evening, our sons were permitted to come to see their new brother. They were not allowed in my room, but I could go with them to see Eric, as soon as I felt like it. I decided I was going with them then, whether I felt like it or not! I wanted to see the reaction on their faces when they saw Eric's head. I was very concerned that they accept him and love him, no matter how large his head was.

David helped me into a wheelchair. Perspiration drenched my body. I felt weak and faint; yet my determination to go to the nursery was strong. Had David described Eric's appearance to the boys before their arrival? I wondered.

As soon as we arrived, Eric was brought to us. My fears subsided immediately when I watched the sparkle in his big brothers' eyes, as large grins broadened across their faces. You would have thought they were looking at the baby who had been voted "most handsome" of all the newborn males.

They couldn't have been any more proud of their new brother. They began to talk to him and call him by name. I wanted to hug David Jr. when he said, "He's pretty. His head's not so big." Again, I felt tears of joy trickle down my cheeks. Shortly, we left and the boys returned home with their grandmother.

Due to my many friends at the hospital, my stay was filled with staff visitors. There was never a quiet moment, it seemed; and excitement added to my exhausted feeling.

The needle in my arm transfusing the IV fluids became uncomfortable. I realized the fluid was infiltrating (running into my tissue instead of my vein). I felt if I called the nurse and told her, she would remove it since I was taking an adequate amount of fluid by mouth. Instead she said, "Well, as soon as this bag goes in, the doctor will probably let us take it out."

It was almost seven o'clock. I knew no one else would be around until shift change. I counted the hours marked on the bag and found I would have to endure about four more hours of fluid running into the tissue of my left arm. After the nurse left, I removed the tape and needle from my arm and ran it into the wastebasket. The nurses still think I just took the needle out when the bag became empty.

For four days my obstetrician kept me on a clear

liquid diet. I still think he was trying to punish me for being so dogmatic about wanting to remain awake for my section. Even with the clear liquid diet and endurance of hunger pangs, I was happy.

Sunday evening, I held to the wall and walked to the special-care nursery. I stayed so long that I'm sure the nurses got tired of me. At 2:00 a.m. Monday morning, I woke up and returned to the nursery for about an hour. At 8:00 a.m. I was there again. By this time, the nurses figured I would pester them to death, so they consented for Eric to come to my room.

It is not hospital policy to permit an occupant of special-care nursery to go to his mother's room. Thus, I became a privileged mother. The nurses emphasized that I should let them know if I became too tired. (That was a laugh! I was past the point of becoming tired, but I wasn't about to let anyone take my baby on that account!)

Every hour or two, a nurse from the nursery came to check on Eric and asked if I was too tired to keep him any longer. I always said, "No."

On Tuesday I went early to get my little one from the nursery. That day the nurses got tired of coming and getting "no" for an answer, so they began calling me on the phone instead. Still, I always said, "No." I honestly believe the afternoon-nursery shift forgot about him. They let me keep him until eleven-thirty p.m.

I began to reminisce. The Friday night before surgery, I had heard the babies being brought to their mothers and thought I would not know the feeling with this baby. Now those mothers only had their babies at designated times, but I kept mine all day long! I enjoyed being the exception. I couldn't see enough of Eric in spite of my exhaustion and hunger!

The neurosurgeon also let me know on Tuesday that Eric's hydrocephalus was the Dandy-Walker type. "We'll let him go home with you and get fatter. I'll want to see him in three weeks, and if all goes well, we'll do his surgery about that time."

Wednesday, I called David and gave him a list of all the baby's homegoing things. I had unpacked them less than a week before, thinking I would have no need for them. The boys were excited that Eric would be coming home with me.

Thursday morning, I informed my doctor that I was ready for discharge. Eric's pediatrician and neurosurgeon had already okayed him for discharge. On the fifth day after surgery, I went home with my baby—a baby who "wouldn't live—and if he did—would be grossly abnormal" . . . a beautiful, live, neurologically normal baby, except for the size of his head.

I honestly wouldn't have traded him for any normal beautiful baby in the newborn nursery. I couldn't see his enlarged head for looking at his beautiful skin color, his dark eyes, and the soft dark hair at the nape of his neck. I saw his beautiful hands with his long, slender fingers clutching my forefinger. I saw the sweetest smiles as he slept. No doubt, he was the most beautiful miracle baby in the whole wide world to me, and I was privileged to be his mother.

Now, I was the mother of three boys. The trial of

Eric's birth had made David Jr. and Brian even more precious to me. As David drove us home from the hospital, I prayed, "Lord, please make me the kind of mother my three boys need. I didn't realize just how precious they were to me, until now. Help me not to fail them."

The name Eric means "hero." Somehow, I knew within myself that Eric would be just that. His miraculous existence alone would show forth God's loving kindness and wondrous works. I didn't care about his being a "hero" for the world, but instead, a "hero" for the One who not only gave him life, but would also heal him.

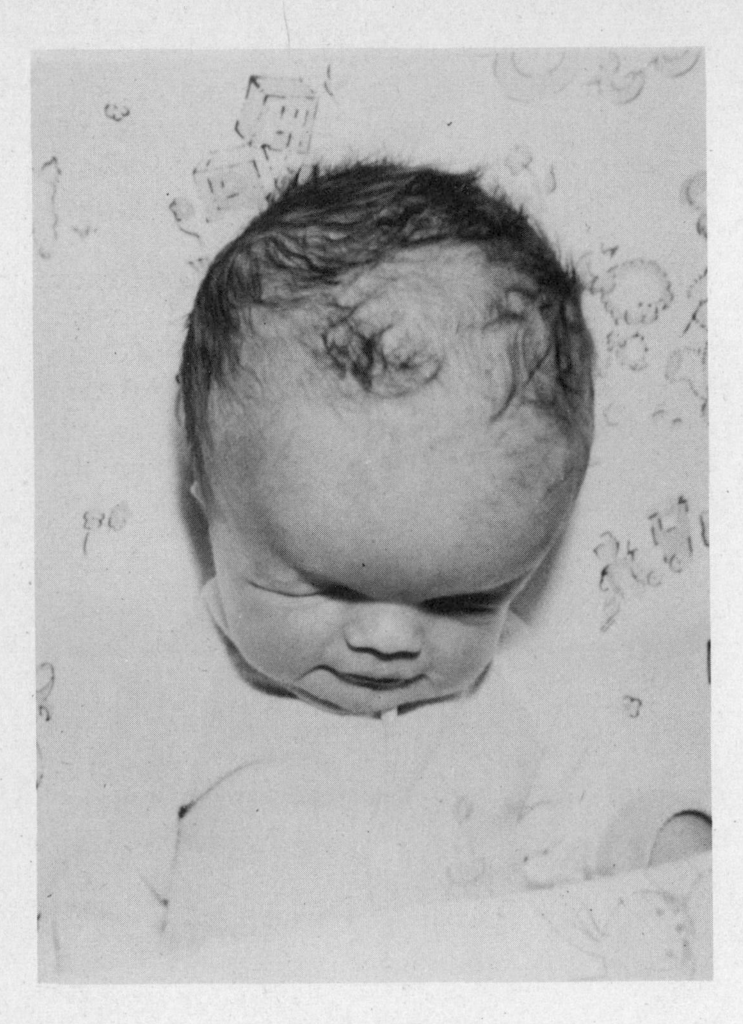

Eric at birth
March 29, 1980
9 pounds, 4½ ounces

6
Curiosity Seekers

During the first few days at home, I could do nothing but count my blessings and bask in the Lord's goodness. Only occasionally would my mind drift to, Why did this happen to my baby. The neurosurgeon had said that Dandy-Walker hydrocephalus was not inherited. "Then what caused this?" I wondered.

The Lord brought three other verses to my attention as I read my Bible. Still in the Psalms, in chapter 103 verse 12: "As far as the east is from the west, so far hath he removed our transgressions from us." In chapter 103:3, "If thou, Lord, shouldest mark iniquities, O Lord, who shall stand?" In Isaiah 43:25, the Lord says, "I, even I, am he that blotteth out thy transgressions for mine own sake, and will not remember thy sins." These verses seemed to reinforce the impression that the Lord had *not* sent Eric as chastisement for past failures. Besides, I thought as I held him in my arms, "How could anything so precious be punishment?"

Just as I had real victory that Eric was sent to me as a blessing for a special purpose, the devil started throwing discouragement my way. It came in the form of curiosity seekers.

The people who had hurt me the worst: the ones who had sought to destroy me with their tongue, the so-called "friends" who turned out to be enemies, and others who never manifested themselves as friends—these heard of my plight and decided to visit me out of "Christian concern." Their motive of curiosity was so transparent; I would have been ashamed to show my face if I were them.

Not only were their motives obvious, their reactions were not in good taste. They would talk to others (word always drifted back to me) expressing how "pitiful" the whole situation and deformity was. It made me sick that grown people could be so foolish. I didn't think Eric was pitiful at all!

Each time my doorbell rang, I received my indiscreet guests graciously. The grace came from above. My flesh didn't want to open the door. The visits I tolerated well; however, I found difficulty coping with some of the remarks.

Eric had been home a short while, and I had endured several of this type of visitor. It was becoming more difficult to answer the doorbell. I knew if I refused to answer the door, they would think I was ashamed of him. Nothing could have been further from the truth! Thus, I continued to answer the door reluctantly. One day I prayed one of those "tell the Lord what to do prayers."

"Now, Lord you've really helped me receive these ignorant, pitiful people. But please, Lord, don't let two particular people come. (I named them.) You've promised not to put on us more than we can bear; and Lord, you know that would be more than I could bear! So please don't allow these two people to visit. Okay, Lord? Amen."

Two days later, the doorbell rang. I was in the back bedroom with Eric. As I approached the door, I could see through the window that it was the very two people I specifically asked the Lord not to allow to come! I darted back behind a nearby door facing, hoping they couldn't detect my moving silhouette.

I began to wrestle with the situation. I thought, "I need to talk to the Lord about this!" I said, "Now Lord, (I should know by now not to begin a prayer with 'Now Lord'!) I'm simply not going to the door! I asked You not to let this happen! Now, here they are to gloat over my situation!"

They reminded me of Job's friends in the Bible. Remember when Job was afflicted, his "friends" came to him and inferred that the affliction was because of sin. In Job 22:5 they asked him, "Is not thy wickedness great? and thine iniquities infinite?" I was determined not to answer the door. This was just too much!

I pondered more verses in the Psalms.

> "Yea, mine own familiar friend, in whom I trusted, which did eat of my bread, hath lifted his heel against me."
>
> Psalm 41:9

> "For it was not an enemy that reproached me; then I could have borne it; neither was it he that hated me that did magnify himself against me: Then I would have hid myself from him: But it was thou a man mine equal, my guide and mine acquaintance. We took sweet counsel together and walked unto the house of God in company."
>
> Psalm 55:12-14

The bitter memories of the hurt and reproach I had borne because of these people began to surge within me. I repeated, "Surely, Lord, You don't expect me to let them in!" I glanced to see if they were leaving. Much to my dismay, they stood persistently at the door.

I remained stubbornly hidden. Then, the Lord seemed to speak to me. He brought another verse to my mind: "If I regard iniquity in my heart, the Lord will not hear me." (Psalm 66:18) The spirit of forgiving overwhelmed me, as the Lord caused me to reflect upon His sufferings for me at Calvary. He seemed to say, "I never sinned; yet they spat in my face, plucked out my beard, beat me until I didn't even look human, and hung me on a cross in naked shame. I still said, 'Father forgive them for they know not what they do.' Now, don't you think you can forgive them?" I opened the door.

There had been many times I had wished for a private moment with them. I would have told them how their attitude and actions toward me almost destroyed me. I wanted to tell them that God would judge them for their hindrance to my life. This was my grand opportunity to tell them, but now that desire wasn't there. I can honestly say with the Psalmist, "I behaved myself as though he (or they) had been my friend(s) or brother(s)."

They only stayed a short while and appeared quite uncomfortable when I could only talk of the Lord's blessings. Did they expect to find a grossly abnormal looking baby with an emotionally distraught mother? I don't know. I only know they never came back.

Curiosity seekers—God's grace was sufficient for them also.

> "But in my adversity they rejoiced and gathered themselves together: yea, the objects gathered themselves together against me, and I knew it not: they did tear me and ceased not. With hypocritical mockers in feasts, they gnashed upon me with their teeth."
>
> Psalm 35:15-16

The devil said, "Lock the door, and don't let anyone else in."

The Lord said, "Let come who may; trust me, and I will be glorified."

> "Fret not thyself because of evildoers, neither be thou envious against the workers of iniquity. For they shall soon be cut down like the grass, and wither as

> the green herb. Trust in the Lord, and do good; . . ."
>
> Psalm 37:13
>
> "Vengeance is mine; I will repay, saith the Lord."
>
> Romans 12:19

Thus, the Lord continued to give me strength to receive those who visited out of curiosity. I still had to fight off the temptation of Satan. I did it by reading the Word of God as I had never read it before. Reading the Bible became more precious to me with each passing day. My love for it grew until I felt I must have it to survive. So when the devil sent discouragement my way in the form of man or circumstance, I would quote scripture verses that the Lord would bring to my mind. I even composed a little chorus I would sing:

> "Keep the devil on the run;
> Use God's word as your Gatling gun.
> His discouragement isn't fun;
> Keep the devil on the run."

7

From Good to Bad

I had almost decided not to return to work. I had become so attached to my precious bundle of joy! However, my mother, a retired Licensed Practical Nurse, had also grown to love Eric very much. She seemed to need fulfillment in her life and informed me she could take care of Eric if I wanted to return to work. So, in about 3 weeks I did return to my nursing position. I knew I would need at least one week when Eric had his surgery.

I would not advise any new mother to return to her job three weeks after a Caesarean section; however, this unwise decision proved to be fruitful. It gave me daily opportunity to have contact with Eric's neurosurgeon, in the event I had questions regarding his condition or care.

Eric progressed well with his growth and development; and at three-and-a-half weeks, he entered the hospital for his shunt operation. The doctor put in a "unishunt." (This is a tube which coils up on the end, terminating in the baby's abdominal cavity. Ideally, it should uncoil as the child grows, preventing the need for multiple replacements because of growth.) The surgery itself went well.

Six days later (just when I was in hopes of taking Eric home) Eric began having petit mal seizures. The left side of his body twitched rhythmically. Although I had observed many seizures during my career as a nurse, it was still frightening to watch my own baby convulse.

He had six or seven seizures that evening lasting from fifteen seconds to two minutes before they were brought under control with phenobarbital. The fontanels of Eric's head became quite depressed, giving Eric an awkward appearance. The doctor reassured me that in time Eric's head would shape up, while his body grew in proportion. Eventually he would take on a fairly normal appearance.

Eric was discharged from the hospital a few days later and remained on phenobarbital. He did well, and I decided to return to work.

A couple of months passed, and I noticed Eric's head shape was not following the doctor's prediction. The front fontanel would be puffed and tense for five days and then become suddenly depressed and remain depressed for six to seven days. When the fontanel was tense, Eric was irritable. When it was depressed his mood and appetite improved.

One day, while at work, I told Dr. Johnson that

Eric's head was not doing as he said it would. He left the impression that sometimes the shunts do work intermittently, but that it may adjust itself. "It's better that it is working some than not at all." He either ignored or avoided my question as to how his head would shape up if it were to be an inconsistent up and down thing with the fontanels.

Toward the end of June, Eric's front fontanel became permanently depressed. His head began to take on a pear-like shape (large in the back and small in the front). His forehead began to narrow, giving his face a rather peculiar shape. He became less social, his appetite decreased, and he would vomit. He began having seizures again. I called Dr. Johnson; and without seeing Eric, he referred me to a neurologist.

When we went to the neurologist, he increased the dosage of phenobarbital and set up an appointment for Eric to have an EEG. If it showed anything significant, I don't know. I never really heard a clear interpretation of it.

Eric continued to vomit and lost weight. Twice, he quit breathing. As his condition worsened, I realized I would have to quit work. I could tell Mother was finding it difficult to cope with his deteriorating condition. I, too, would lose sleep, checking often to see if he were breathing and desperately trying to keep him nourished, in spite of his vomiting.

Finally, I purchased an apnea monitor from a respiratory-care supplier. This little device permitted Eric to sleep on a sensitive pad, placed just under his mattress. It would cause a beeper to alarm if Eric should quite breathing for longer than ten seconds. This was a lifesaver for both of us. It brought me badly needed sleep and could startle him enough to make him breathe if he did stop.

I really believe that he was a prime candidate for Sudden Infant Death Syndrome (crib death). I continued to manifest my concern to Dr. Johnson when he passed through our unit. I was beginning to wonder if he really wanted Eric as a patient. I thought maybe he was too busy for my baby.

One afternoon, I talked at length with the neurologist to whom he had referred me. He seemed quite concerned, but helpless as to Eric's needs. I had a picture made of Eric and brought it to work. When Dr. Johnson came through the unit, I showed him Eric's picture. He seemed more concerned, but did not seem to think there was any reason to rush. He simply suggested I bring Eric to see him in September (this was late July) as we had planned. During the time we waited to keep our appointment, Eric's seizures became more frequent.

Finally, on September tenth, a brain scan was done that revealed that the enlarged cyst was not draining; it was only increasing in size. The shunt had been placed in Eric's lateral (side) ventricles, not in the enlarged cyst. This accounted for the caved-in appearance of the front of his head and the enlarged back of his head. Dr. Johnson said he would call me when he decided what to do.

I waited for a week to hear from Dr. Johnson. Each time my phone would ring, I expected it to be him. When it wasn't, I would rush the caller off the phone—"In case the doctor tries to call . . ."—I would say.

I had quit work on August twenty-ninth; so, I was unable to talk with him as he passed by. I was desperate! My calls to his office were fruitless. Finally, I called my former head nurse and asked her to please question Dr. Johnson regarding Eric, hoping the very mention of Eric's name would serve as a reminder for him to call me. I was convinced he had forgotten my son existed!

When she asked him about Eric, he expressed that his surgery wasn't an emergency. I was furious! Maybe it wasn't an emergency to him, but it was to me! If it were his baby vomiting and having seizures, he'd change his opinion!

I was tempted to call him and tell him I was going to let him babysit Eric on his next weekend off. I would like to have watched him attempt to keep Eric nourished and clean him up for twenty-four hours.

Eric could successfully manage to mess up everything within three feet of any location in which he vomited. Not only would I have to wash his clothes, but mine. I had to shampoo the chair I held him in, and the carpet—eight to ten times a day! This became almost routine.

Approximately one week went by before I finally talked with the doctor. It so happened he had to go out of town; but he reinforced the statement I had heard second-hand: "This is purely elective surgery, not an emergency."

In spite of my anger, I respected Dr. Johnson. He was known as one of the best in our vicinity. As far as I was concerned, he was the best. I felt I must trust his judgment. I asked the Lord for guidance and strength to endure the time which lapsed between that day and the day when Eric would be scheduled for surgery.

On October 15, 1980, Eric was finally admitted to the hospital for his second shunt operation. The night before surgery, Dr. Johnson took me into the nurses' office in the pediatric unit to talk with me. I could tell by the expression on his face that what he was about to discuss would not be pleasant.

He began, "You know when Eric was born, I mentioned that along with his Dandy-Walker hydrocephalus, he had agenesis of the corpus callosum?" (underdevelopment of the membrane which lies in the center of the brain and transmits impulses to the different hemispheres in the brain). I nodded affirmatively. He continued, "Well, now I do not think he has a corpus callosum at all. This probably means there will be some mental deficiency, possibly more severe than we had initially thought. To be honest, I really don't know to what degree it may affect him.

I said, "I understand." There was a pause. I think he anticipated that I would be tearfully upset. Instead, I said, "You just operate on this little fellow like you would if he were yours. Do a good job. He may be operating on your head some day! If Eric should be retarded, then God will give me grace and strength to face that when it becomes evident, but I really don't think he's going to be."

He said, "Okay," and left.

I returned to Eric's bedside. His roommate was a darling four-year old Dandy-Walker hydrocephalic boy who had been admitted for a shunt revision. He looked perfectly normal and manifested perfect intelligence for his age. Ironically, his mother was also a registered nurse who had worked as an emergency room nurse throughout her pregnancy.

Earlier that afternoon, it had been such an encouragement to watch him. Now, I began to wonder what Eric's outcome would be. I also became concerned with the treatment Eric would or would not receive in the future. I had watched other doctors "throttle back" on treatment of those who had dim prognoses of "being productive individuals." I did not want this to happen.

I advocated doing all that could be done for him, except putting him on a breathing machine to sustain his life. If it came to that, I would draw the line. The past month had been agony.

Dr. Johnson had not been aggressive enough to suit me. Now he seemed to have reason not to be "over-zealous" in his treatment, if he shared the same views as other doctors I had heard talk. He had stated when Eric was born that he felt "doctors should do their best for babies like Eric." Did he still feel this way? I prayed that he would. I'm sure he thought I had not reacted very realistically to his news of Eric's corpus callosum not being there at all.

The reason this sad piece of news did not drive me to tears was because the Lord brought a verse to my mind that I had read only a few days before bringing Eric to the hospital.

> "The Lord will perfect that which concerneth me; thy mercy, O Lord, en-

> dureth forever: forsake not the works of thine own hands."
>
> Psalm 138:8

I knew when I read the verse that God was able to make Eric perfect without doctors. I prayed desperately that the Lord would cause the enlarged ventricle to drain without surgery. I asked Him to make the necessary opening it needed. He did not see fit to do it as I requested; therefore, I felt He had chosen to use Eric's neurosurgeon to accomplish this task. (*If* Dr. Johnson would let the Lord use him, I thought now!)

Dr. Johnson decided to leave the shunt in the side of Eric's head, as well as put a new one in the back to drain the enlarged back ventricle (or cyst). This sounded okay. However, I couldn't help but wonder why the shunt wasn't put in the back the first time. When I asked, Dr. Johnson said it was the usual procedure to shunt the side first. This was my first indication that Eric was not the typical Dandy-Walker hydrocephalic baby. He was not responding well to the usual corrective surgical procedure.

When the front fontanel depressed and remained so, Eric's growth and development began to regress. I knew that he had shown potential for being normal; however, the neurosurgeon had not witnessed it.

He seemed to look questioningly at me now when I referred to the things Eric had formerly done. He had been able to hold a rattle, to play with his hands, laugh and coo aloud; in fact, the main things he had trouble with were focusing his eyes and holding up his head.

To me, it was understandable that these two tasks would be difficult due to the accumulation of fluid; especially since we now knew that the fluid pressure in the back of his head had never been adequately relieved.

He also showed signs of having trouble with his equilibrium. With any sudden movement, he would grab with his hands, hold his breath momentarily, and then cry as if he thought he were falling. Cuddling him closely and stopping the movement would calm him immediately. "Often when he's on his back, with the slightest movement, he acts as though he thinks he's falling," I would tell the doctor (an over-reactive startle reflex is the way I interpreted it medically).

The doctor never offered any explanation for this problem. As his vomiting and seizures became more frequent, Dr. Johnson seemed preoccupied with other things. I knew I had obtained the best neurosurgeon in the area, but I was becoming annoyed with him.

Should I have permitted Eric to be sent to the other hospital as most hydrocephalic infants were? This and other questions began to haunt me. Would his treatment be as agressive now that Dr. Johnson felt he might be mentally or physically retarded? Was this why he had waited so long to do the shunting operation? Was he hoping that I would be content to just leave Eric alone and watch "nature take its course"? The old saying "actions speak louder than words" was beginning to manifest itself with him. I did not like what I saw.

Eric's second shunt was placed into the back of his head on Friday morning, October seventeenth. Eric did poorly after his surgery. He came back very congested. A cool-mist vaporizer was ordered for him. It drenched him as well as his bed linens moments after it was directed toward him. I was convinced if he didn't have pneumonia, he would shortly acquire it!

After his surgery, Dr. Johnson visited him, but to me he seemed more evasive when I asked questions. I knew he felt I was avoiding reality. His associates visited Eric and totally evaded my questions. I wondered why they even came by. They were never any help.

Eric had great difficulty retaining anything he took by mouth. He began projectile vomiting worse then ever before. The attempts to keep an intravenous needle in his tiny veins were practically hopeless. He became very weak when I could only get him to retain four to eight ounces of clear liquid in twenty-four hours.

I experimented with thickened feedings and practically every kind of baby formula, including goat's milk and yogurt. Absolutely nothing worked! Eric soon refused to suck a bottle at all. Then I made frantic attempts to keep him hydrated by dropping into his mouth two to three treaspoons of clear liquid every thirty minutes, all day as well as all night long. Needless to say, I became physically exhausted.

Any attempts made by the nurses to start an intravenous line proved to be fruitless. Eric was now retaining only four to six ounces over a twenty-four hour period.

The next day Dr. Johnson's associates came to visit Eric. I begged them to do a cut-down (cutting the skin and putting an intravenous needle directly into a visible vein) so that Eric could at least get enough intravenous fluids to enable me to take a rest from my frantic attempts with a dropper. His associates passed the buck by saying, "That's up to Dr. Johnson."

"When will I see him?" I asked.

"Probably not until tomorrow."

"Then would you write an order for a nasogastric tube?" (This would enable the nurses and myself to give him fluids through a tube passed from his nose to his stomach.)

"Not without Dr. Johnson's permission."

They left, and I became more furious with every passing second. For three days and nights now, I had kept my baby alive with a drop at a time of pedialyte (a clear liquid electrolyte solution). No one seemed to care about the fact that he wasn't having an adequate intake and, consequently, was losing weight.

My angry meditation was interrupted when one of Eric's former nurses from special-care nursery came in to see him. When I told her of Eric's long struggle and of the predicament we now found ourselves in, she replied, "I would've already been in a psychiatric hospital, if this had been my baby; I wish you would've let him go to the other hospital. I feel they would've put forth more effort for him over there."

After she left her words, ". . . I wish you would've

let him go to the other hospital. . ." still lingered with me. Did I make the wrong choice when Eric was born? I was exhausted both physically and emotionally; and quite honestly, it seemed impossible to think logically about anything.

Feedback from those closest to me indicated their feelings that perhaps someone else should see Eric. Now Eric's former nurse expressed the same opinion.

I needed God's direction. My head throbbed so badly I found it impossible to read my Bible. I wept, then made a long overdue decision to face Dr. Johnson and his associates with my feelings.

I called down to the operating room and talked with one of my friends who worked there. She informed me that Dr. Johnson was in surgery. I called two different units in our hospital where Dr. Johnson placed most of his patients. His associates were not in either unit; therefore, I decided to begin my search on the first floor of the hospital.

I found Dr. Johnson's nurse in the emergency department. I asked her where Dr. Carter (fictional name for one of Dr. Johnson's associates) was. She indicated he was treating a patient and asked why I needed him.

I began, "I am very upset with the care Eric is receiving. I'm sick and tired of Dr. Carter refusing to make any decisions on Eric's behalf. Eric must have more intake than he's had the past few days if he's going to live! It seems at the moment none of his doctors care whether he does or not. If Dr. Johnson has more important patients to attend, then all he needs to say is that he's too busy for

Eric. I'll be more than happy to take him somewhere else. In fact, if I don't hear from Dr. Johnson shortly, I will leave this hospital with my baby and his records; and you all won't have to be bothered with him anymore." *It is a patient's right to obtain their records and seek other medical attention, when they feel the attention they are receiving is inadequate. Parents may do this on behalf of their child.*

She promised she would deliver the message to Dr. Johnson. I went back to Eric's room and waited impatiently. A few hours passed. The door opened. Dr. Johnson, his nurse, and Eric's pediatric nurse entered.

Dr. Johnson took a seat as he pulled a chair close to where I was sitting. He began, "Now—what is it that you feel we are not doing right?"

"I just think you're too busy for my son. You must have felt sorry for me the day I asked you to take him as your patient in the intensive-care unit. I think you consented to care for him out of the goodness of your heart." (Dr. Johnson was a well-known, highly respected neurosurgeon. He didn't need patients. His services were sought after for miles around.)

I rambled on, not giving him a moment to defend himself from my verbal attack. "Eric needs medical attention. He isn't keeping enough nourishment to live. Sure, he's hydrated; but it's only because of the efforts I'm making. I can't stay up another night dropping fluids into his mouth every hour. He needs an intravenous line desperately. Dr. Carter visits your patients, but he acts as though he can't make any decisions. Now, the nurses are unable to get an intravenous catheter into Eric's veins. Do you want to try? Why do you hesitate to do a cut-down?" I ran out of breath (for which I'm sure he was grateful) and paused.

He very calmly began to reassure me that he wanted Eric as a patient. He explained that the hazard of a cut-down (which I already knew) was a new "portal of infection."

He continued, "If Eric's skull does not shape up on its own, then plastic surgery will be in order." (Cranioplasty surgery, in which the baby's skull would be taken apart surgically and re-shaped). "This surgery is a very bloody procedure; therefore, Eric will need all the good veins we can find in order to get needed blood. If I do a cut-down, that vein would not be able to be used in a few months if we needed it. Let's give Eric a few more hours, before we consider a cut-down seriously. Try to calm down, and don't do anything desperate."

I consented reluctantly, and they left.

I began to pray—"Dear Lord, I'm about to fall over. No one seems to understand. I can't keep going twenty-four hours a day. What do you want me to do?" He seemed to say, "You've been trying so hard to do everything yourself. Why don't you let Me take over?"

I began to cry, realizing how foolishly independent I had become over the past few days. Oh, I had prayed often, saying, "Lord, help him to eat," or "Lord, please don't let him vomit this ounce." But in my desperate attempts to care for him, I had neglected my Bible miserably. No wonder my stength was failing; I had not been drawing from my Source. As I read in Psalm 86, joy and peace were once again my comfort:

> ". . .For thou art great, and doest wondrous things: thou art God alone . . . O turn unto me, and have mercy upon me; give thy strength unto thy servant, and save the son of thine handmaid. Shew me a token for good; that they which hate me may see it, and be ashamed: because thou, Lord, hast holpen me, and comforted me."

Moments later Eric began to suck his bottle, as I held him in my arms. By eight o'clock that evening, his liquid intake totaled more than it had any day since surgery. Thus, it wasn't necessary for me to sit up and drop fluids in his mouth every hour. I slept deeply on the cot next to his bed that night, rising only once to feed him. I felt a refreshing renewal of strength.

It was several days before Eric was released from the hospital. His vomiting persisted, but his intake was adequate enough to keep him hydrated. I was giving him total care, but I missed my other two boys very much. I asked Dr. Johnson to discharge Eric by stating, "I can do the same things at home that I'm doing here."

He agreed and discharged him, even though he was only averaging around six ounces intake in a twenty-four hour period. He seemed confused as to the reason for Eric's continuous vomiting.

This was the second indication I had that Dr. Johnson either did not know what else to do or was not going to do a lot more. I had given him the opportunity to refer me to someone else, but he had reassured me that he wanted him as a patient. Why, then, was he not more concerned with Eric's nourishment?

I could not figure out his motive. If he did not know how to help Eric further, why would he not refer me to a neurosurgeon who specialized in children's neurosurgery? How could I be sure that Eric's problems weren't related to his digestive track? I questioned this possibility, but my concern was ignored.

I took Eric home with so many unanswered questions.

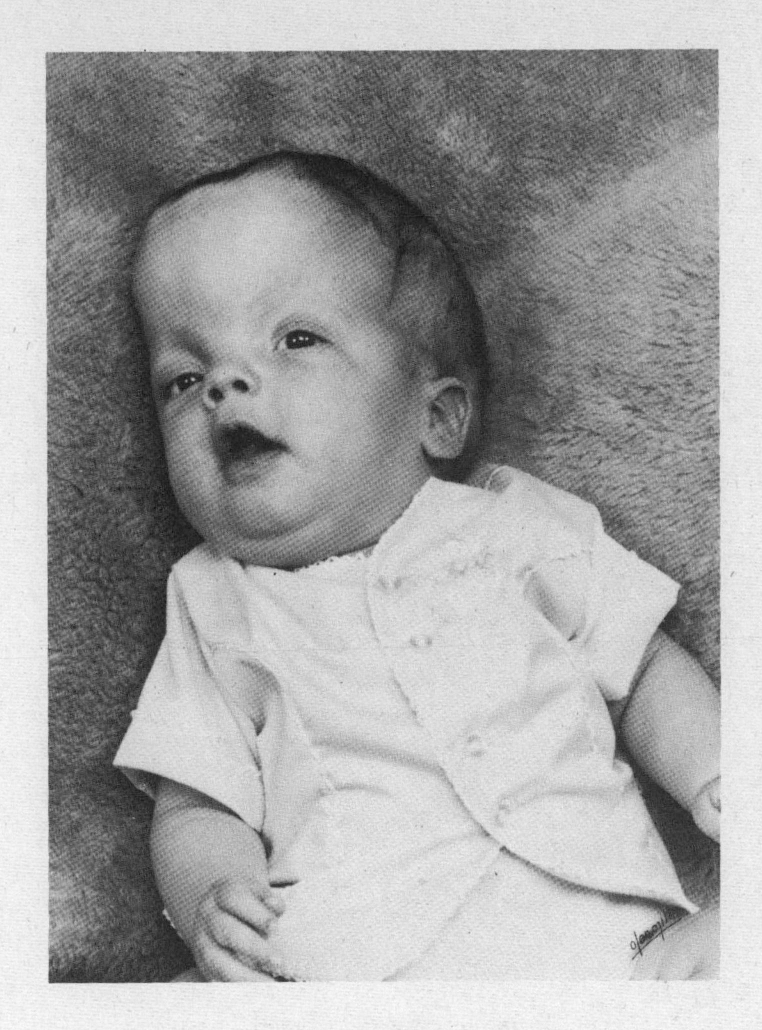

Eric, 3 months
17 pounds

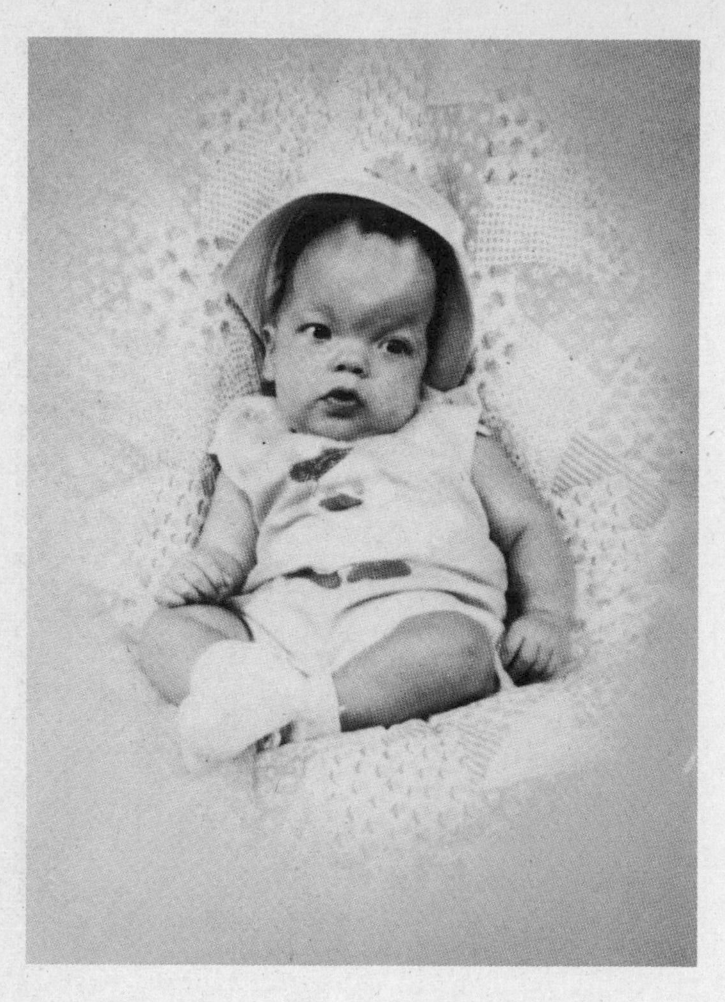

Eric, 3½ months, Anterior fontanel depressed

8
From Bad to Worse

Temporary improvement came with Eric's homecoming. His pediatrician put him on medication for his equilibrium, which seemed to help his nausea for a few days. Then Eric resumed his deteriorating course.

With Eric's noticeable weight loss, I observed that his muscles were wasting away and that he was not moving his right arm or leg. I began exercising both arms and legs with more emphasis on the right side. He became less alert with every passing day. When I exercised him or attempted to push nourishment on him, he would fuss weakly as if to say, "Mommy, leave me alone!"

While he was awake, I made sure every waking hour was filled with stimulation. I read the Bible and sang to him.

His head was so out of shape and had been shaven so much, that one of my favorite songs was my revision of "Jesus Loves the Little Children." It went like this:

"Jesus loves the little children,
All the children of the world.
Red and yellow, round and square,
He even loves those without hair.
Jesus loves the little children of the world."

I played cassette tapes of reading of the New Testament, remembering Proverbs 4:20-22—"My son, attend to my words; incline thine ear unto my sayings. Let them not depart from thine eyes; keep them in the midst of thine heart. For they are life unto those that find them, and health to all their flesh." He could listen, absorbing the Word of life. Besides, it was refreshing to me to listen while folding diapers or caring for him.

His room was filled with brightly colored toys and objects he no longer noticed. He lay lifeless. The only way I could get him to smile was to whisper the name "Jesus." I wondered now if I were being selfish in wanting him to live. He seemed to be drifting so close to Heaven.

The verse I had clutched so often came to my mind: "The Lord will perfect that which concerneth me . . ." I began to wonder now if He intended to make Eric perfect on earth or in Heaven.

I had watched Eric suffer so much. Perhaps I was being selfish in wanting Eric to stay with me. I opened my Bible and began to read, thinking, "Okay, Lord, if you're going to take him, I'm going to need some strength."

Much to my surprise, the Lord didn't lead me to Psalm 23 or to 1 Thessalonians 4:13-18. Instead I read:

> "Wilt thou show wonders to the dead? Shall the dead arise and praise thee? Selah. Shall thy lovingkindness be declared in the grave? or thy faithfulness in destruction?"
>
> Psalm 88:10-11

Again, he gave me peace that Eric was going to live. I began to thank him for all He had done for me through Eric's crises. I felt such peace and joy from reading His word. I thought of how unworthy I was to feel His presence so near and sweet. In Psalms 91:4 I read, "He shall cover thee with his feathers, and under His wings shalt thou trust: his truth shall be thy shield and buckler."

It was such sweet communion with my precious Lord that I began to say, "Lord, what can I do to show You I love You?"

He called to my remembrance, "I thought you said you didn't want to do anything except be a bench warmer at church."

"I remember, Lord, but I'm sorry. I'll do anything You tell me to do. But Lord, I can't even take Eric out now; he's so sick. I can't imagine what I could do, except be a good wife and mother. I've been so stubborn; I'm surprised You'd even consider using me for anything."

Then He brought to my mind Isaiah 64:8—"But now, O Lord, thou art our father, we are the clay, and thou our potter; and we all are the work of thy hand." He seemed to say, "It's not the old Jennifer

I'm going to use; it's the new one I've made."

"Well, Lord, I'm willing; but I'm scared. I want You to show me very plainly what You want me to do. I don't want to jump into anything that isn't Your will," I replied.

Once again, His word was His answer:

> "Trust in the Lord with all thine heart; and lean not unto thine own understanding. In all thy ways acknowledge him, and he shall direct thy paths."
>
> Proverbs 33:5-6

As I pondered the fact that a potter couldn't mold clay until it was soft and with a shape of its own, I scribbled this tune on a nearby piece of paper:

> "Je-sus changing me,
> Yield-ed I shall be,
> Je-sus break-ing,
> mold-ing,
> mak-ing,
> Je-sus changing me."

Two days later, our associate pastor's wife called and said the Lord had laid it on her heart to ask me to speak at the next Ladies' Fellowship Meeting at our church. I was afraid to say "no," and I graciously accepted.

Our church attendance averaged approximately 2,800, and I began to get a little nervous wondering how many ladies would be there. I had never spoken before a group of women in my entire life. The Lord calmed my fears and assured me He would give me the words to say.

A few days before the meeting, Eric began to get

worse. Again, I had to resort to dropper feedings of clear liquids, every night and day. I was becoming exhausted again; and quite frankly, I began to wonder what I was going to praise the Lord about at the meeting!

Earlier, when I was exuberant with the Lord's blessings, I thought I had my talk ready. When I realized that I was about to let circumstances defeat me, I became more determined to give God praise and glory in spite of my exhaustion and Eric's poor condition.

The meeting was held, and David fed Eric while I was away for approximately two hours. The Lord blessed the meeting and gave me some of the sweetest friends I have ever been privileged to know. From that time forth I was showered with the support, love, concern, and prayers of God's people such as I have never witnessed in all my church-going years. I realized God had taken from me the people who were not best for me and replaced them with His "jewels."

How defeated I would have been while encountering this crisis with Eric, if I had remained in my former circle of friends! I could not grasp the warmth and love of these ladies. *I never knew such love existed among Christians!*

Shortly after the meeting, I took Eric back to Dr. Johnson for a post-operative check-up. I told him Eric was still vomiting. He replied, "I don't understand why he has this vomiting syndrome. Maybe in time it will resolve itself. I don't know what else to do."

I asked if there were a children's gastrointestinal

specialist that I could take Eric to in order to rule out any digestive problems. He did not seem to think it was a digestive problem. His conclusions were less than satisfactory to me.

In the course of our conversation, he asked if I were depressed a lot and kindly told me to call him before I "took any desperate action." (By this I assumed he meant to call him before I decided to make an attempt to locate another neurosurgeon!) "Call me at home anytime, if you need to," he concluded.

I left his office with an empty feeling. The best neurosurgeon around just admitted he did not know what else to do for Eric! He didn't feel that Eric should see a GI specialist, but I could call him if I needed him.

Eric continued to vomit. On Thursday, November 13, 1980, I obtained the name of a pediatric GI specialist from a friend of mine at a nearby hospital. I called the specialist and described Eric's diagnosis and condition to him and begged him to see Eric. He very graciously consented and on the next day accompanied Eric to the pediatric X-ray department for an upper and lower GI X-ray.

The X-ray revealed a slight esophageal reflux, but he determined that it should not be causing Eric's continuous vomiting. His concern and compassion were exactly what I needed, and the X-ray did rule out several other problems that could have caused a "vomiting syndrome." Eric and I endured the weekend.

The following Monday I took Eric to his pediatrician. He could find no infection or reason for his continuous vomiting but commented, "You're doing a good job keeping him hydrated. The only thing I can suggest is to take him back to Dr. Johnson."

That evening I called Dr. Johnson. "Do you want to see Eric, or do you want me to take him somewhere else? He's actually starving before my eyes!"

He concluded that he would like to re-admit him to the hospital the following day.

On November 18, 1980, Eric was a patient in the hospital once again. That afternoon, Dr. Johnson came into Eric's room and sat down. He began, "The only other thing I can think of to do is to remove the shunt in the side of Eric's head. Perhaps we are draining too much fluid with two shunts. Maybe this is causing him to vomit. There is a high risk, however, that after the shunt is removed, fluid accumulation in the ventricles may increase his intracranial pressure so rapidly that it could take his life before anything could be done to reverse it. You decide what you want me to do. It is a decision you'll need time to think about. If you decide on the surgery, we can plan it for Thursday or Friday."

There was a pause; then I spoke. "Well, he can't go on living like he is. It would be more merciful for him to die suddenly than to gradually starve to death." He nodded, agreeing with my rationalization. I continued, "I just don't understand. He did so well his first three months. I can still get a smile out of him occasionally.

Dr. Johnson said, "Yes, but you want a better

baby than that."

I nodded with reservation. What did he mean by that statement, I wondered?

"If it would make you feel more comfortable, we could call for a second opinion," he said suggestively.

I agreed that it would make me more comfortable.

I was just about to talk to the Lord about this situation when nursing supervisors began to enter. Obviously, they weren't as interested in Eric as they were in me. When their concern was directed quite pitifully toward me, I realized immediately that they expected Eric to die.

I suppose they had heard I had a decision to make. Eric could die slowly or quickly, depending upon my decision. After all, if the "very best neurosurgeon" doesn't know what else to do, Eric must be written off as a lost cause.

The "poor Jennifer look" on their faces was all it took to depress me to tears. I lost my composure, and for a while I lost all the faith I had. I felt like God had forsaken me. With my crying, I developed an intense headache. I would no more than dry my tears and attempt to rest on the cot beside Eric's bed, when more nurses would drop in with sympathetic looks.

The tears would begin all over again. I felt almost like a grieving mother beside her baby's casket. No one, absolutely no medical person was even giving Eric the benefit of a doubt! He was doomed to die! The nurses were coming by to see how I was taking the situation. I guess they were wondering if I were still "hung up" with denial, or if I had finally accepted the fact that I was going to lose him.

Down deep, I still did not believe he was going to die (still clutching to denial); however, I found myself playing the part of acceptance real well. I just wanted them to leave me alone.

My head was throbbing. I felt alone in my fight to save him, and I didn't have the strength to argue my side. Finally, I was able to sleep a few hours while my headache subsided.

Around midnight, I was able to read my Bible in the quiet of Eric's room. It was like looking at my soul through a mirror as I read:

> "I am weary of my crying: my throat is dried: mine eyes fail while I wait for my God."
>
> Psalm 69:3

> ". . . In the day of my trouble I sought the Lord; my sore ran in the night, and ceased not; my soul refused to be comforted. I remembered God, and was troubled: I complained, and my spirit was overwhelmed. Selah . . . Thou holdest mine eyes waking: I am so troubled that I cannot speak . . . I call to remembrance my song in the night: I commune with mine own heart: and my spirit made diligent search. Will the Lord cast off forever? and will he be favourable no more? Is his mercy clean gone forever? Hath God forgotten to be gracious? hath he in anger shut up his tender mercies? Selah."
>
> from Psalm 77

In subsequent chapters I read of the miracles God performed for the children of Israel. He seemed to reassure me that He was still a God of miracles: the same yesterday, today, and forever. Then once again he reminded me to put my trust in Him as I concluded my reading with Psalm 84:11-12:

> "For the Lord God is a sun and shield: the Lord will give grace and glory: no good thing will he withhold from them that walk uprightly. O Lord of hosts, blessed is the man that trusteth in thee."

I drifted off to sleep with peace in my heart that Eric would live.

The next day, another neurosurgeon from a nearby hospital came to see Eric. I watched him quietly examine Eric neurologically. After he finished, I asked him what he thought. He put me off by saying he would have to see Eric's brain scans before giving an opinion on him. It seemed logical enough. "I'm going to look at them now," he said as he departed.

I waited some time for his return. Impatiently, I walked to the nurses' station. I noticed he had left his belongings there, so I knew he had not left the hospital. Shortly, I saw him return. I returned to the nurses' station to ask him again what he thought. He stated that he wouldn't be able to tell me anything until he first spoke with Dr. Johnson. I replied, "Okay," and walked back to Eric's room somewhat disgusted.

I began to ponder the fact that the hospital CT scan room is ordinarily closed over the weekend. If Eric's surgery were to be done on Friday, and if he began to show signs of increased intracranial pressure over the weekend, it would be difficult to get a brain scan done in a hurry. I was concerned about this possibility.

I knew that Dr. Johnson could put in a ventricular drain or a reservoir that could be tapped immediately if Eric's pressure began to increase rapidly. It was my impression that Dr. Johnson was planning to make this one last attempt; and if it didn't work, then—goodby, Eric! I wasn't ready to give up!

When some of the nurses came in to visit, I discussed my thoughts with them. (That was a mistake!) I guess they expected me to still be in tears over the fact that Eric was going to die (they thought!). They looked at me rather leerily and commented that as good as Dr. Johnson was, I could be sure that he would know what was best for Eric.

Since I had regressed into the denial stage of grief, they didn't stay around long. After all, they realized quickly that I didn't need their sympathy. I had received a new portion of comfort and strength from the only One who could make Eric well. This was comfort, I'm sure, that they did not understand.

In nursing school, all nurses are taught the stages of grief. If a family does not follow these stages just as the book states, then they will probably need psychiatric counseling. What was worse, I was a nurse. I should not only know the "stages," but should be normal and quit being unrealistic.

Dr. Johnson was in surgery and did not visit Eric,

making it impossible for me to discuss my thoughts with him. I pondered the idea of this safety-valve option with the reservoir or the ventricular drain all day long. It seemed like a good idea to me. It would be better to have it and not need it, than to need it and not have it!

I realized I was not going to have peace of mind until I talked to Dr. Johnson. I was afraid he would not come by the next day before Eric's surgery. Periodically, I kept in touch with a friend who worked in the operating room in an attempt to talk with the doctor after he finished surgery. As it happened, he had a long, hard day (probably not finishing until after 7 p.m.). He managed to leave the hospital without my getting in contact with him.

I felt reluctant to call him at home because I knew he was exhausted; however, I felt I must speak with him. After all, he had told me earlier to call him at home if I felt it necessary. Therefore, I decided to call him.

He was short and indifferent to me as he spoke, reiterating the fact he had gone through a long day in surgery and would talk with me in the morning. He made me angry.

I thought to myself, "He only has occasional twelve-hour work days. I worked regular twelve-hour days during the nine months I was pregnant with Eric. Many of those days were spent struggling to keep that doctor's patients turned to the position he so dogmatically emphasized they should be!"

I felt that he had not meant his suggestion that I

should call him! "Phooey on him!" I said aloud as I jerked the sheet across my cot.

After I lay down, I felt ashamed that I had allowed myself to become so furious. At least I would be able to talk with him in the morning. That was some consolation.

Along with the morning sun came Dr. Johnson into Eric's room. The sun was by far the more cheerful of the two! I could detect by his facial expression that he was still annoyed with me. He expessed the fact that he had gone through "a long day yesterday and didn't get much sleep."

I quickly rebounded. "Don't tell me about not getting sleep. I haven't had an uninterrupted eight hours' sleep in over a year now!"

He could tell that I was not in a cheerful mood myself. We both became more understanding of each other as our conversation began. I told him of my desire to have a drain or a reservoir on Eric.

He explained that a ventricular drain would not be a wise choice because of the risk of infection. Then his ego began to expose itself as he spoke in his typical stern manner.

"Why don't you take care of your other two sons and your husband; and leave this type of decision up to me, since I am the one who's been trained to make them!"

I quickly defended myself. "I am taking care of my other two sons and husband, but we have all grown accustomed to Eric's face and we don't want it to be absent from us just yet!"

Tearfully, I continued, "I'm afraid you're giving up on him after this surgery. I wonder if you would even call for a scan for Eric over the weekend, since you feel he's going to be retarded anyway. (Only emergency cases are scanned on the weekend.) Would you deem Eric an emergency if he needed a scan?"

He answered he would, and continued—"And if I decided to put in a Rickham reservoir on Eric and he lived, I want you to understand that it would not be the result of your thinking up a new procedure!" I felt like spitting.

Raising my voice slightly, I said, "I'm not TRYING to 'think up' a new procedure! I'm simply trying to grasp at one other alternative! You said that if this didn't work, you did not know what else to do. I'm trying to buy time. I still believe that something can be done to help him!"

He replied that the other neurosurgeon had agreed that he should take this planned course of treatment. (In other words, the other well-respected neurosurgeon didn't know "what else to do" either. Finally, I was hearing the second opinion, secondhanded!)

"I still would feel more comfortable if you would put in a Rickham," I said persistently.

As he got up to leave, he mumbled that he would "consider it."

Most highly successful doctors do not take kindly to women questioning their judgment and are even more insulted when nurses make suggestions to them. I could tell I had "ruffled his feathers"! I was sorry that he was upset; nevertheless, I was glad that I had made my feelings known.

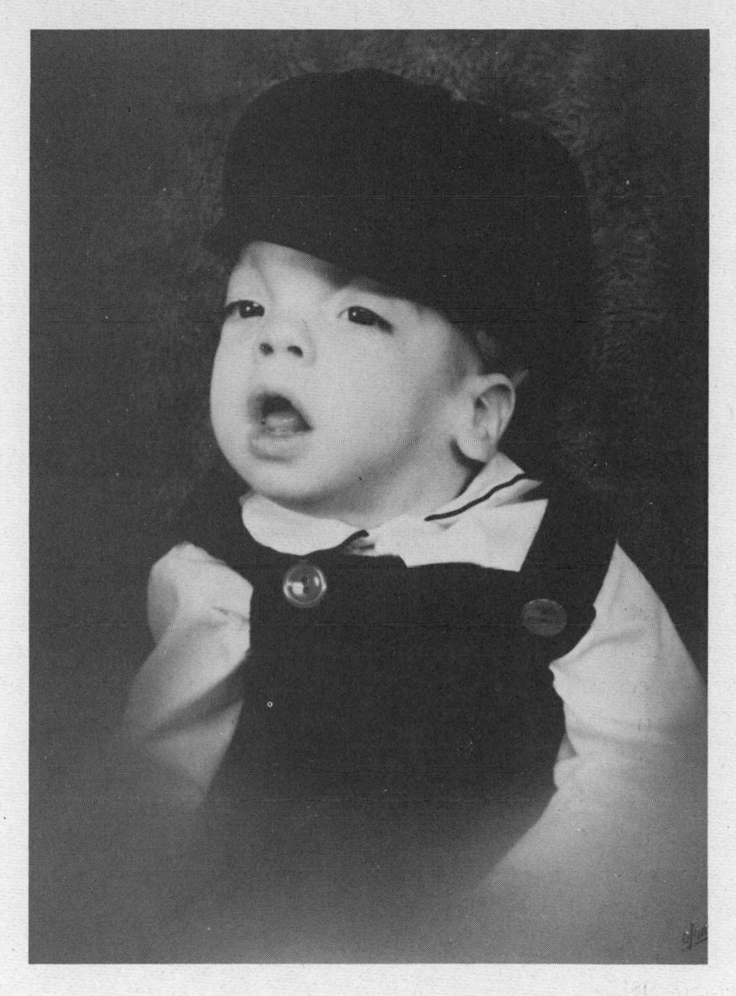

A hat conceals Eric's deformity and surgical scars. We never hesitated to have portraits taken when his condition enabled us to do so.

9

"Lord, Nobody Cares"

During Eric's surgery, Dr. Johnson did place a Rickham reservoir in the place where he removed Eric's first shunt. Post-operatively, however, Eric continued to vomit periodically. He seemed to have one good day, tolerating good amounts of clear liquids; and the following day, his "vomiting syndrome" would return.

I got the definite impression that Dr. Johnson would not pursue Eric any further. I decided to phone the doctor who came to see Eric from the other hospital. Perhaps he would pursue Eric's case a little further.

I felt something had been overlooked and God had the answer waiting for us somewhere. Perhaps I should consider transferring him to the other hospital.

That idea was quickly removed from my mind as I spoke with the other neurosurgeon by phone. When I asked if he could recommend a children's neurosurgeon, he replied, "I don't know of anyone else who would do any better by him than the surgeon you have. I feel the baby has a poor prognosis." (In other words, he did not feel Eric would live either.)

I persisted, "What about a children's hospital somewhere? Is there not one you could recommend?"

He seemed annoyed with me now as he replied, "If you take that baby anywhere else, you're going to be losing the interest of all the neurosurgeons in this area, and that's exactly what you have here. I don't know anyone else that I would recommend."

I thanked him for his time and hung up the phone. For a split second it sounded nice that Eric had the interest of "all the neurosurgeons in the area." Then I realized that all their interest wasn't doing a thing for him! I began to wrestle with the idea of taking him somewhere else.

Shortly, one of Dr. Johnson's associates came in to visit Eric. I mentioned to him that I wanted a children's neurosurgeon to see Eric. He, too, was annoyed with my idea. Very bluntly and rapidly he spoke, "You want a second opinion? I'll give you a second opinion. Any other doctor will tell you to take that baby home and love him until he dies. Most neurosurgeons would have never operated on that baby to start with. His brain isn't normal!"

He spoke with such emphasis, as if he were trying to get it through my thick, stubborn mind that Eric would not live regardless of where I tried to take him!

"Take him anywhere you want to go . I'm sure Dr. Johnson won't mind," he continued.

"Where would be the best place to take him?" I asked.

"I don't know!" he said very disgustedly as he left the room.

"It's almost impossible to get another doctor to see a patient without a referral," I thought as the tears began to flow once again.

I cried for at least an hour after the doctor left, as I reminded the Lord that He promised His grace would be sufficient for me (II Corinthians 12:9). Right then, I didn't feel His grace, and I couldn't understand why.

Again, several nurses came to visit. (The loyalty of nursing supervisors to doctors is amazing!) Now, they didn't come out of concern to me. They made it clear that I was making a mistake to even entertain the idea of taking Eric elsewhere.

"You're a nurse. You should know if our doctors can't help him, then no one can. We've got the best here!" they bragged.

One supervisor went to another floor and discussed Eric and my reaction with personnel there. (It was very unethical for her to discuss Eric's case off the unit. As a nurse, I was taught that this was considered "betrayal of confidence.")

Word came back to me that she had stated that she was surprised at me—that I should take him home and love him until he died and accept the fact that he could not live.

Another supervisor told a friend of mine (in a location other than the hospital) that being a nurse, I should be more realistic—that I should not be "grasping at straws," hunting for other medical attention.

Not only were these nurses unethical, but indiscreet. I felt I was not only battling doctors now, but nurses as well.

All this lack of concern and understanding came my way the day before Thanksgiving. That night as I lay awake on the cot, I again asked the Lord why I didn't feel His sustaining grace.

Again He impressed upon me to pick up my Bible and open it to read. These are the verses that stood out in my mind as I read:

> "God is our refuge and strength, a very present help in trouble. Therefore will we not fear . . . Be still and know that I am God."
>
> from Psalm 46
>
> "In God have I put my trust: I will not be afraid what man can do unto me."
>
> Psalm 56:11
>
> "Be merciful unto me, O God, be merciful unto me: for my soul trusteth in thee: yea, in the shadow of thy wings will I make my refuge, until these calamities be overpast. I will cry unto God most high; unto God that *performeth all* things for me."
>
> Psalm 57:1-2

> "Give us help from trouble: for vain is the help of man. Through God we shall do valiantly: . . . "
>
> Psalm 60:11-12
>
> "My soul, wait thou only upon God; for my *expectation* is *from him.*
>
> "God hath spoken once, twice have I heard this; that *power belongeth unto God.*"
>
> Psalm 62:5 and 11

He told me through these verses why I had not felt His sustaining grace. I realized I had taken what the doctor had said as imminent fact. God had told me earlier on different occasions that Eric was going to live. Now, one blunt opinion from a doctor threw me for a loop!

I became so upset when my faith failed in the face of testing! I was angry at myself for putting my confidence in man. The Lord wanted me to be totally and completely dependent on Him.

Just to be sure that I understood what the Lord was trying to tell me, I asked Him to "Shew me a token for good" (Psalm 86:17) if he really were going to make Eric well—I asked Him to help Eric to keep some kind of milk. I had tried everything and was at my wit's end as to what to try next.

Again, the Lord used my neighbor Frances in a miraculous way. Shortly after I had read and prayed, I talked with her by phone. She suggested that I try Eric on sweet acidophyllus milk. She even offered to go look for some and bring it to me.

I said, "Let me first check with dietary here to see

if they have it."

I hung up the phone and called dietary to inquire about the milk. They had a small amount and would send it up for Eric. That evening he began taking sweet acidophyllus milk and did not vomit. I was so excited!

The next morning I got up early to pray and read. What I had thought was to be the worst Thanksgiving of my life turned out to be the best. God had heard, God had answered; and, what's more, God would heal! How—I did not know!

It became more apparent to me with each passing day that He would not use Eric's doctors in His plan, unles they changed considerably. I was still baffled as to where I should go.

As I read my Bible I kept seeing these words:

> "O my God, I trust in thee: let me not be ashamed . . . Yea, let none that wait on thee be ashamed: . . . O keep my soul, and deliver me: let me not be ashamed; for I put my trust in thee."
>
> from Psalm 25

I said to myself, "No one should ever be ashamed that they have put their trust in the Lord."

He seemed to put me to a test and say, "Well, since you feel that way, re-emphasize to Dr. Johnson that you're trusting Me to heal Eric."

Then my thoughts drifted back to yesterday's comments: "She's a nurse . . . she should realize that he can't live . . . Take him home and love him until he dies . . . If our doctors can't help him, nobody can!"

I knew how well-respected Dr. Johnson was. He

was highly revered by the nurses. When he spoke, they jumped! They had a holy fear of displeasing him. I figured that since I had already been labeled by nurses as unrealistic, I may as well let Dr. Johnson assume that I was a religious fanatic as well.

Moments later, I read Psalm 26:7—the verse that motivated the writing of this book: "That I may publish with the voice of thanksgiving, and tell of all thy wondrous works."

Just before noon, Dr. Johnson arrived as I had started out the door with Eric; we ran into each other.

"Happy Thanksgiving," I said cheerfully.

"Happy Thanksgiving to you, too." He looked at Eric. "I hope that some day we can wish him a happy Thanksgiving and that he'll understand."

"Don't worry; we'll be able to. Listen, I know you don't know anything else to do for him, but the Lord has told me that he's going to live. I'm writing a book about him, and the last chapter isn't going to be his funeral!" I rattled on.

He and the nurse in charge were silent for a moment. Then Dr. Johnson spoke, "I see he's done well with his fluid intake."

"Yes, he has," I answered.

"Well, we will just have to take a day at a time with him and see what happens," he said as he walked toward the door. After he left, I wondered for a split second just what he thought of my statement.

Of all the health-care professionals I had to deal with, the only ones who seemed understanding were the pediatric nurses. They were jewels!

The head nurse told me one day to do exactly what I felt I had to do. "You're going to have to live with the decisions you make regarding Eric. Do whatever you feel you can live with," she said.

They were supportive and genuinely compassionate during each of Eric's hospitalizations, but they could not ethically give advice and direction. Only the Lord could direct me; thus, I resigned myself finally to leaning completely on Him.

I began to wonder if He were going to heal Eric in spite of doctors, or because of them. I knew He could do either.

The Saturday following Thanksgiving, Eric was discharged from the hospital with little comment except to "Take a day at a time, and call me if you need me," Dr. Johnson stated briefly. Eric had been in the hospital on Brian's birthday and on Thanksgiving Day. I wondered momentarily as we left the hospital where we'd be at Christmas.

Brian and David Jr. had decorated the house for Christmas to surprise me when Eric and I came home. On Saturday evening, Eric began to vomit again; however, he did retain enough so that I was able to sleep six hours on Saturday night.

I knew that if God did not see fit to perform a miracle soon, Eric would not live until Christmas. My faith wasn't weakening; I was simply getting impatient for the Lord to work. I wanted others to see Him heal my baby speedily! In fact, I wouldn't mind seeing Eric well for Christmas!

Sunday morning after David and the boys left for church, I sat in a rocking chair beside the Christmas tree holding Eric. As I was thanking the Lord for the two little boys who had decorated it and for the one in my arms, I began to be concerned with the fact that I probably wouldn't be able to buy David, David Jr., and Brian any Christmas presents. "Besides," I thought, "by now everything must be picked over."

Just for a moment, it bothered me; until I noticed a shining gold ball. In the ball, I saw the reflection of Eric and myself. He was lying sweetly asleep on my shoulder.

I penned these words on a paper close by:

"Reflection of a Christmas ball
Glistening on the tree,
As I hold my baby dear
Oh so close to me,
No Christmas package could compare
With this moment that we share.
Just to be together here
Is gift enough dear Lord from Thee."

Again, tears of gratitude began to flow as I mediated on God's blessings in my life. I thought of His birthday and wished I could give Him something special for Christmas. I pondered just what I could do to let Him know how much I loved Him.

On previous Christmases David and I had been able to give in special offerings at church. With my being unemployed and with Eric's medical expenses, that would not be possible this Christmas. I said, "Lord, surely I could give something; tell me, Lord, what could I give to let You know how grateful I am for Your lovingkindness and blessings

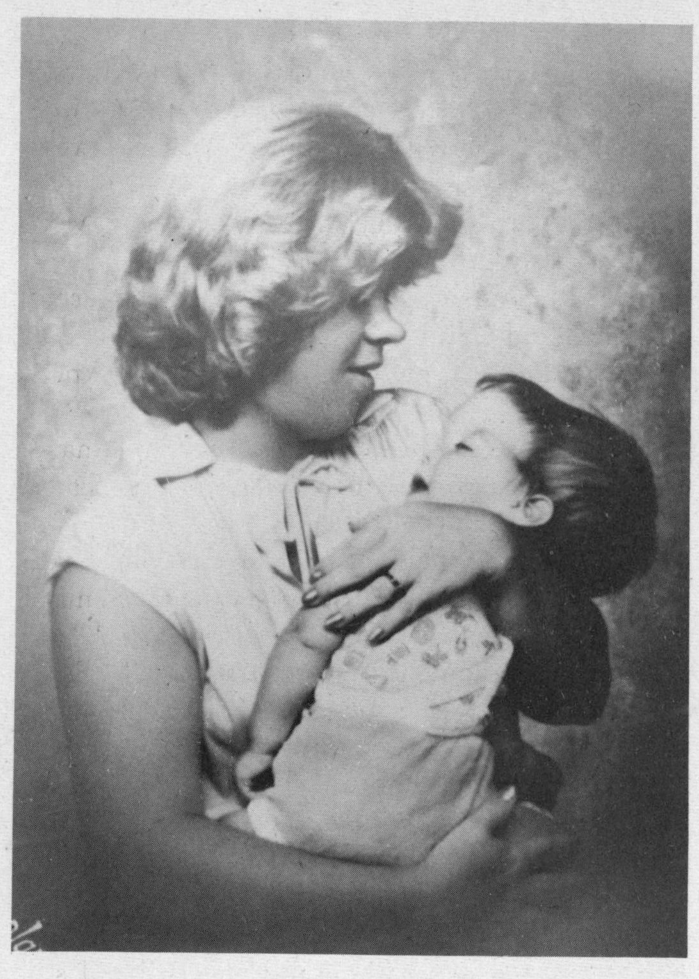

" . . . No Christmas package could compare with this moment that we share . . ."

on me?"

It was almost as if He were sitting in my den talking with me. I love to feel this near to my precious Saviour; but, surprisingly, our conversation went something like this:

"You'd really like to show Me that you love Me?"

"Yes, Lord, You know I would."

"You sure do love that little fellow in your arms, don't you?"

"You know how much I love him! You know how precious he is to me!"

"Why don't you give him to Me for Christmas?"

"Why, Lord, You know he's Yours. I dedicated him to You when he was born."

"That wasn't exactly what I meant. Since you dedicated him to Me at birth, then you won't mind Me calling him home at Christmas, will you?"

"What?" (My heart seemed to skip a beat.) "Surely You don't mean—but, Lord, You've promised me that You were going to let him live! I've already gone out on a limb and told people You were going to heal him! All the medical people think I'm a religious fanatic now. Why, I'll be the laughing stock of the hospital, if You take Eric to heaven!"

"People laughed at Me, and mocked Me, and I could have called ten thousand angels; but I still died for you! I suffered persecution for your sake. Could you not suffer a little for Me?"

"Yes, Lord, but—"

"I never promised you how long I would let him live. Why, if I took him today, he's already served a purpose in your life."

"I know, Lord, but—"

"But what? The truth is, you love him better than you love Me."

I was so ashamed. Weeping bitterly, I said, "No Lord, I'm sorry. I do love him, but not more than You. Take him. He's Yours. He always has been. As much as I'll miss him, he'll be happier with You, I know. Thank You for lending him to me for these precious few months."

By now I was crying so that I couldn't say any more. I wept for several minutes before I realized Eric was resting so quietly against my chest. I quit "snubbing" enough to check him to see if he was still breathing. I thought, for a moment, that the Lord had already taken him. He was breathing.

"I guess, Lord, that You're going to wait until Christmas to take him. I wonder what time it will be? Could You sort of slip him away quietly, perhaps, while he sleeps? It's hard to watch him suffer, Lord."

There was stillness as I began to wonder if I should try to prepare David and the kids for Eric's homegoing.

"There's no use in doing that," the Lord seemed to interrupt my thoughts; "I'm not going to take him."

"What did you say, Lord?"

"I said, I'm not going to take him."

"But, Lord, if that's what You want, I said You could have him."

"That's what I wanted. I wanted to see if you loved Me enough to give him to Me. I'm satisfied that you were willing."

I was overjoyed; once again my faith was renewed

in such an unusual way. I felt as though I knew what Abraham must have felt as he offered up Isaac.

A couple of weeks passed, and I took Eric to Dr. Johnson for a check-up. My faith was so strong that as soon as Dr. Johnson had looked at Eric, I began to chatter boldly about the fact that the Lord had promised me in Psalm 138:8 (quoting it for him) that He was going to heal him. "I know the medical outlook for him is bleak; and I know you think I'm stuck in the denial stage of grief, but I'm telling you that Eric is going to be a case for the medical books! He's going to be completely well! Perfect! The Lord has promised me so!" (By now, I'm sure he would have liked to have found a soap box for me to stand on!)

He said that he would do his best, and the rest was up to God. But he said it with reservation, as if I were expecting more from God than he was. He advised me to leave Eric flat, hoping to deter some of his vomiting episodes.

On Christmas day, I felt as though I were taking a cold. When I took care of Eric, I wore a mask over my face. His resistance had to be low.

As I sat holding Eric at the table, he raised himself into a sitting position on my lap, as if to say, "Merry Christmas, Mommy." I was so thrilled I forgot all about feeling bad! He sat up twice again on Christmas evening. Each time he smiled, I was so excited!

My joy soon turned into worry as Eric got sick the day following Christmas. My mask evidently had not served its purpose. By now, I knew that it wasn't just a cold, but the flu instead.

It was all I could do to care for him; and as he became worse, so did I. I called his pediatrician.

"Oh my g-o-s-h!" he said.

There were people in a lot better physical shape than Eric who were dying with the type flu we had. In fact, I was so sick that I rather expected to die myself! I just couldn't manage to fight it off.

My own lack of sleep and failure to take care of myself over the past year had caused my own resistance to fall to zero. I don't remember ever feeling so bad.

Eric would not take any food or liquids. He would just lie and moan weakly with every exhaling breath. I asked the pediatrician for permission to use a nasogastric tube (a tube passed through the nose to the stomach where fluids can be passed through to supply nourishment) to feed him. I also asked for some antibiotics. I knew that antibiotics would not help the flu, but perhaps it could prevent Eric from getting pneumonia, which could easily follow the flu, especially since Eric was suppose to lie flat.

Dr. Davis was kind and understanding. He okayed the use of the nasogastric tube and sent him a prescription for an antibiotic.

Most doctors would have required that I bring Eric for an office visit, but the weather was icy and cold.

Dr. Davis had always treated me kindly when I would suggest strongly that I felt Eric needed something specific. If he questioned my judgment, he was never arrogant, but was always kind and would explain why my idea was not the best idea.

Several times he would say, "I don't know," and he would be willing to permit me to try something different with him. It was easy to respect the doctor, because he respected me.

While Eric had the flu, I worked with him vigorously. Every two hours, night and day, I would give him chest postural and drainage therapy (positioning him across my lap, his head lower than his body—patting all sides of his rib cage, loosening secretions which may have accumulated in his lungs—then gagging him with a suction syringe, causing him to cough up large amounts of thick mucous).

I would listen to his lungs with my stethoscope. If his breath sounds were not clear, I would repeat the procedure until I could not detect any congestion. I would suction out his nose and mouth and then pour two ounces of liquids through his tube.

I was still feeling rotten through all these efforts. One night I prayed and asked the Lord just to take Eric and me both on to heaven, "Then we'll both be out of our misery," I told Him.

My mother, bless her dear heart, came over and stayed three days to help me. Consequently, she came down with the flu. In spite of our suffering we all survived, and after about two-and-a-half weeks began to see some improvement.

Eric continued to show signs of increased intracranial pressure. His eyes twitched rhythmically more often now. He continued to have petit mal seizures, and his vomiting was still a problem.

Around the middle of January, I took Eric back

for a visit to Dr. Johnson. I expressed my concern over Eric's symptoms of intracranial pressure. He said, "He's just washed out from the flu."

"Then you don't think he needs a brain scan?" I asked.

"No," he replied; and I left his office again very discouraged.

By the latter part of January, Eric's vomiting seemed impossible to control. It was more projectile now. I would feed him three ounces of clear liquid, and it looked as if he would vomit back four as it gushed a couple of feet.

One Sunday evening I called Dr. Johnson and strongly suggested that I felt Eric should have a scan. He promised he would have his office set up one.

A week went by before the scan was done. It was obvious they weren't in any big hurry. I asked the technicians if I could take the scan by Dr. Johnson's office. They consented for me to do so only after they had taped them shut very conspicuously. "If they think a little tape is going to keep me from looking at these, they're crazy!" I thought to myself as I opened them and held them up to the window in Dr. Johnson's office before handing them to his receptionist.

I could see that the fluid build-up was more than it had been in Eric's last scan. I knew that the shunt was obviously not doing an effective job. I was confident that Dr. Johnson would phone that evening to tell me Eric would need a shunt revision. I knew Eric was becoming a high surgical risk due to his already poor, weakened condition.

To my surprise, Dr. Johnson did not call. Several days went by before I was able to get in touch with him. Much to my amazement, he stated that he felt Eric's shunt was draining.

"That's the last straw!" I thought as I hung up the phone. "I know I must get someone else to see Eric." I prayed, "Lord, where would you have us to go?"

I recalled talking with Dr. Davis concerning the possibility of a children's gastrointestinal specialist looking at him. He had given me the name of a doctor who practiced in a university hospital approximately eighty miles from our home. I knew if I took Eric to see that doctor, he would call in a neurosurgeon to see Eric as well.

"This may be the answer," I thought. "Is this what you want me to do, Lord?" I asked.

I asked the Lord if He did not want me to seek help elsewhere to help Eric show improvement. I knew I needed to obtain all Eric's records from the hospital as well as his scans and X-rays before attempting to carry him to another doctor.

That night and most of the following day it snowed, making it impossible for me to make a trip to the hospital for his records. After the snow stopped falling and I could see Eric becoming worse, I decided to go after his records.

I obtained his scans and X-rays from the X-ray department and his records from the medical record department. Of course, I received some rather hostile looks and reluctant cooperation, but I got what I went after. *It is every patient's right or the right of an immediate family member to see and have their own medical records.*

I also went by Dr. Johnson's office for copies of Eric's records there, explaining to his receptionist that it was necessary for my own peace of mind to have someone else see Eric. She was very understanding and cooperative.

The road was extremely slick as I made an effort to return home. It took me *an hour and a half to travel thirteen miles*; but the Lord protected me, and my trip was uneventful.

After I looked over all of Eric's charts, I phoned the doctor at the university hospital. He was not there (naturally), and the operator gave me his home phone number.

Upon reaching his home, his wife said he was out of town for a week, but that his associate would be glad to talk with me. She proceeded to give me his home phone number. I called him.

After explaining a brief medical history of Eric and his present poor condition, I asked if he would consider seeing Eric. Talking about doctors' egos—I was exposed to a whopper this time!

"Lady, (I had given him my name; nevertheless, he did not use it) we don't deal with parents over the phone. We take patients from doctors' referrals, not from parents' requests. If you want to see us, you'll have to get your pediatrician to send us a letter of referral."

I had already explained that Eric was critical and that I was calling long distance. I decided that as long as I had him on the phone, I could be just as persistent as he could be inconsiderate.

"Man, I told you that my pediatrician suggested I

talk with your associate! He gave me his name, and he's out of town. Now, my pediatrician cannot refer me to you when he doesn't even know you exist! If I bring Eric with his records to the university hospital tonight, would you be kind enough to see him?" I asked.

"Even if you were to bring him tonight, we would not have a bed for him. You'd just have to take him to a motel somewhere until we had some discharges, and there's not likely to be any over the weekend with the bad weather." He spoke rapidly, as if he didn't have time for me.

"Then, in essence, you're refusing to see Eric?"

"I can't believe out of the hospitals you have there that someone can't help you," he said, ignoring my straightforward question.

"I told you that doctors from both hospitals have seen Eric and that they don't know what else to do for him. Now, if you don't want to be bothered with him, tell me."

He began to soften a little as he said, "I'll have my office call you Monday and set up an appointment for you. Meanwhile, if you feel comfortable using the nasogastric tube, you may try Vivonex or Progestimeal with him. These are more nutritious with more caloric value. If he can tolerate acidophyllus milk at all, he can tolerate formula."

I thanked him and hung up. Somehow, I doubted if these were the people who should see Eric. I doubted even more that I would ever hear from his office, so I simply said, "Lord, if that's where you want Eric, open the door—if not, keep it closed."

The doctor's office receptionist never phoned. I assumed this was clue enough that Eric would not be a patient there.

Four or five days passed. Eric became worse with every passing day. Not one pharmacist or medical supply place had or had ever heard of Vivonex or Progestimeal, at least not any that I was able to contact. Therefore, I kept him hydrated on acidophyllus milk and clear liquids.

I began to realize that no one cared about even trying to help Eric. He was hopeless and helpless as far as doctors were concerned.

I was physically and emotionally exhausted. I knew I could not continue to exist and neither could Eric, unless God saw fit to do something fast.

I knew what the Psalmist meant now when he wrote:

> ". . . their soul is melted because of trouble. They reel to and fro and stagger like a drunken man, and are at their wit's end."
>
> Psalm 107:26-27

I tried to fulfill my duties as a wife and mother. I could not even think straight, because I had lost so much sleep! I knew that it must be time for the Lord to work.

I prayed, "Lord, you know what a mess we're in. Unless you guide and give wisdom, Eric will die."

> "Hear me speedily, O Lord: my spirit faileth: . . ."
>
> Psalm 143:7

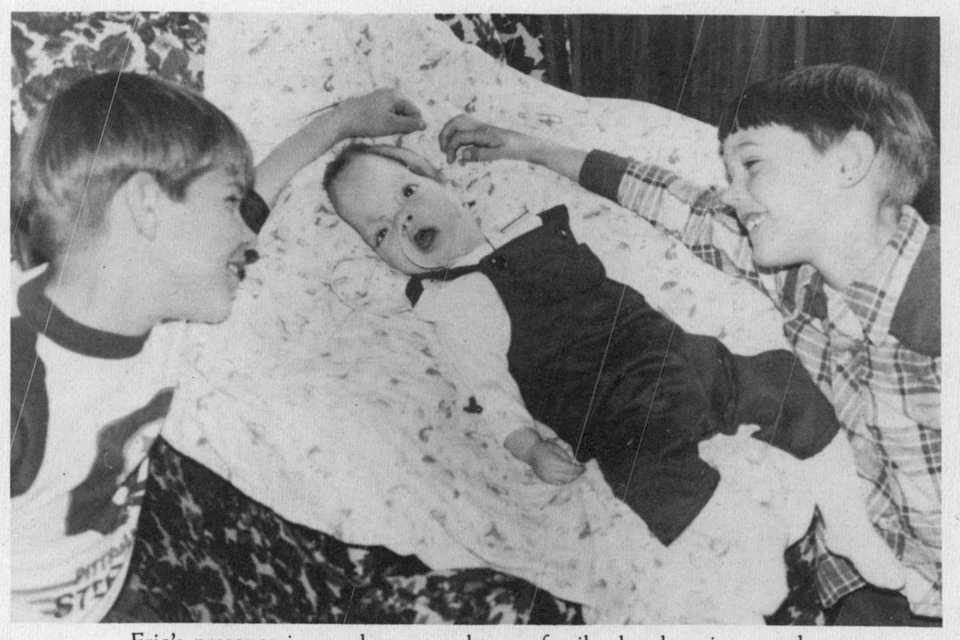

Eric's presence in our home taught our family that happiness and contentment came not from material gain, but from a close relationship with God and with each other.

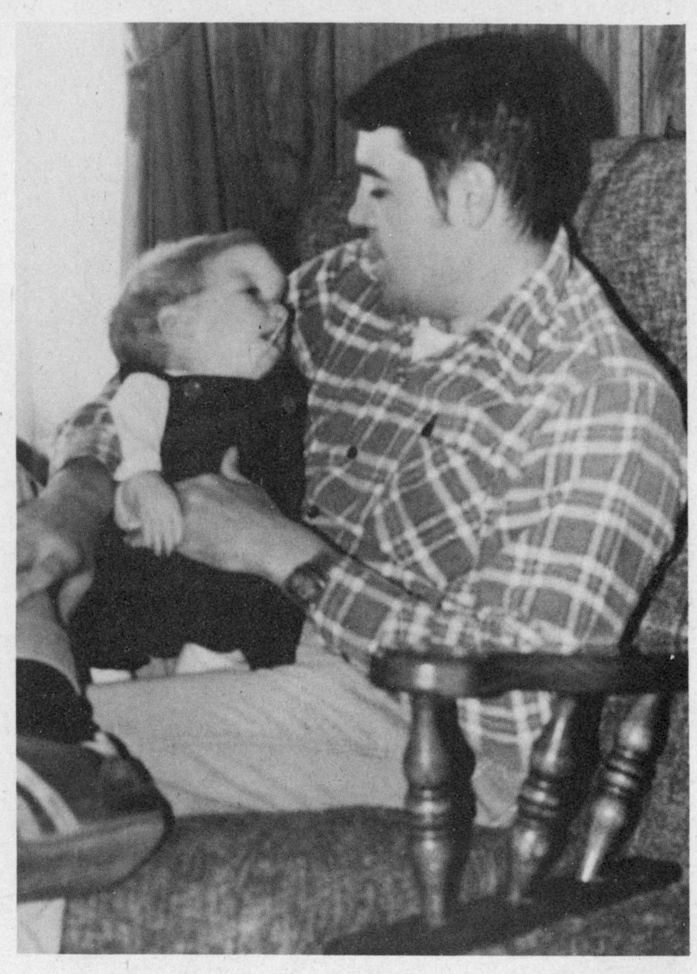

Eric and Daddy

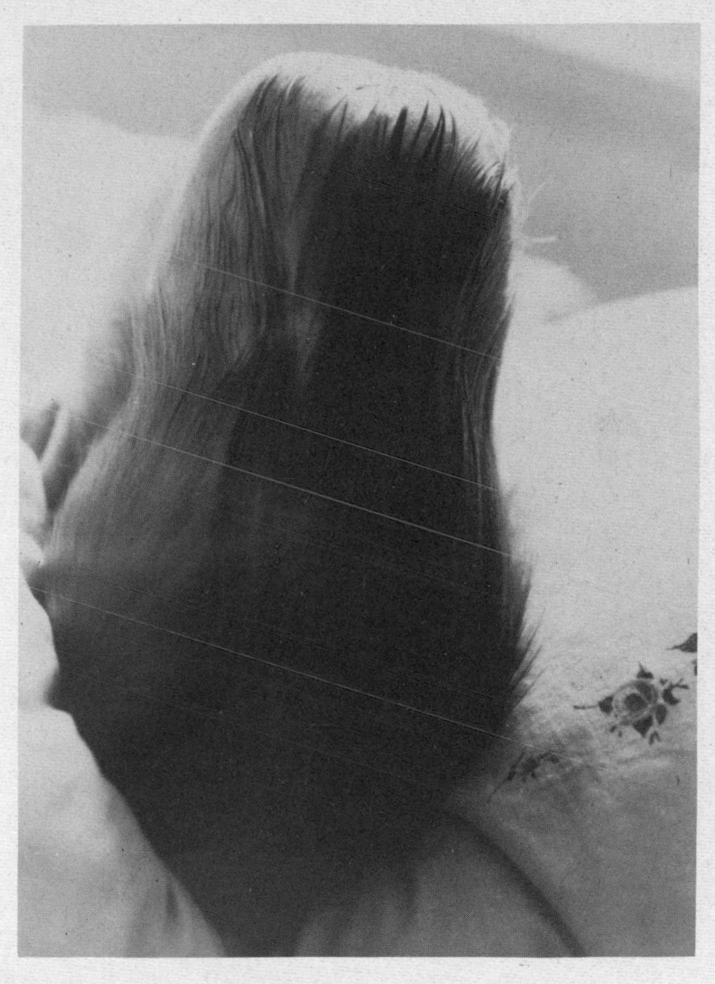

The pear-shaped appearance of Eric's head began to improve after his surgery at Philadelphia.

10
New Direction

On Wednesday night, February 11, 1981, Eric began to show severe signs of intracranial pressure. He cried all night. Nothing I tried to do seemed to help.

He could no longer retain an ounce of clear liquids each hour. I had to very slowly give him one-half ounce an hour in order for him to be able to retain it. He began to arch his back backward in what medical people refer to as an opisthotonic position.

I still knew that the Lord was going to intervene for him. I never once wondered if he were going to live this time. I did wonder to whom the Lord would direct us.

I knew before I took him to anyone else, that I must have Dr. Davis rule out any infection process. An ear infection or a temperature could cause an increased intracranial pressure in Eric.

As the morning sun began to peep through the curtains in the bedroom, I began to count the minutes as I waited for Dr. Davis to get into his office. At eight o'clock, I phoned and asked the receptionist if I could bring Eric in that morning.

"Sure," she answered.

After Dr. Davis examined him, he rolled back from the examining table on his stool and looked at me with a baffled, concerned look. "I can't find any signs of infection. I think the problem is with his head."

I began, "Well, Dr. Davis, I'm through with the neuro people in this area. You know, as well as I do, that he is not going to live if I don't get some help for him. They've admitted they don't know what else to do for him, yet they refuse to refer me anywhere else. I have to seek help elsewhere! I've got to know I've done my best regardless of the outcome. Surely, you must have heard of a children's hospital somewhere that I could take Eric. You read medical journals. Where would you take your child if he were like that?"

He listened with a studied expression; and when I finally paused, giving him a chance to talk, he answered—"I really don't know, but I could put you in contact with someone who may be able to help you. I have a little patient who was born with an open spine. His parents were missionaries, and he was treated at a children's hospital. Just a minute," he said as he left the room.

I noticed as he returned that he had a patient's records. He proceeded to tell me what hospital and neurosurgeon looked after the little boy and then added, "And he's doing real well. I'll tell you what—I'm sure his mother wouldn't mind talking with you about his care. I'll give you her number and let you call her."

I felt like hugging him! I hurried home from his office and got Eric situated as comfortably as possible before I phoned the lady.

Her name was Kitty. She was so kind and understanding. She told me about her little boy Stephen briefly; and then added, "But I was referred to a particular hospital. Even though Stephen received good care there, if I would've had my choice, I would have chosen the Children's Hospital at Philadelphia."

"Why?" I asked.

"Because the chief surgeon there is a Christian. From the articles I've read that he's written, he believes in doing the very best for even hopeless patients. Just a minute—" she said as she left the phone momentarily to find one of his articles.

I was so excited as I waited for her to return. She had already sold me on the idea of contacting him. If he were a "Christian" and believed in attempting to help the "hopeless," then surely he would be kind enough to at least talk with me about Eric.

She returned to the phone. "His name is Dr. Everett Koop, and he's at the Children's Hospital of Philadelphia."

"Thank you so much! I'll try to get in touch with

him," I said hurriedly.

"Jennifer," she said as she stopped me from saying 'Goodbye,' "would you let me know what you find out?"

"I sure will," I said. "Thank you again!"

I placed a person-to-person call to Dr. Everette Koop at the number I had gotten from information. The person who received the call at Philadelphia said, "Just one moment—" with a distinctively Northern accent. I glanced at the clock and noticed it was around lunch time. Butterflies played tag in my stomach as I waited impatiently.

Doubts fluttered through my mind. What if I couldn't reach him. Being surgeon-in-chief there, he might be too busy to talk with me. If I get the same kind of reaction that I received from the other doctor I called last week, I'll just croak!

Two minutes seemed like an eternity before a voice spoke in my ear, "This is Dr. Koop."

I fought tears of anxiety as I began, "Dr. Koop, I'm Jennifer Vanderford. I'm familiar with some of the articles you've written . . ."

"Yes," he said.

"Well, I have a little hydrocephalic ten-and-a-half-months old baby boy who is going to die if a miracle doesn't happen."

I proceeded to give him a brief medical history of Eric.

"The doctors here (I named both neurosurgeons who had seen Eric) feel his prognosis is poor and have admitted they don't know what else to do. Would you all consider looking at Eric there at

Children's?"

He mentioned that he was familiar with the neurosurgeon who had been called in for a second opinion on Eric. He knew that he was highly respected. "However," he continued, "we don't give up on those kinds of babies up here. Even with his agenesis of the corpus callosum—if the hydrocephalus is managed, he could still be fairly healthy. I don't do this type of surgery anymore; however, we have the best children's neurosurgeon in the nation right here. Let's see—"

There was a pause. Then he continued, "Mrs. Vanderford, (he remembered my *name* from my introduction! I was impressed!) I can't transfer your call to his office from this telephone. Let me have your full name again; spell it for me—and your baby's name."

I spelled them slowly.

"Listen, I'll go right down to Dr. Schut's office and tell them you're going to call at my suggestion. His name is Dr. Luis Schut, S-C-H-U-T, and his number is . . ." (He gave me the number, pausing periodically to allow me time to write.)

"Thank you so very much!" I said.

"Now—give me about twenty minutes, so I can go down and tell them about Eric before you call," he continued.

"Okay," I agreed.

We said "goodbye" and as I hung up the phone, I burst into tears as I realized God had directed me to someone who cared. As exhausted as I was from being awake more than twenty-four hours, I still felt like a mountain had suddenly been lifted from my feeble shoulders.

I could not believe the courtesy that this "surgeon-in-chief" exhibited to a frantic, distraught parent. I'm sure he had enough to do without talking to a stranger by phone about her sick baby. If he were busy, he never acted too busy for me.

He talked to me with the warmth and concern a father would use when giving advice to a daughter. His kindness was overwhelming. It was hard for me to believe now that there were some surgeons still left who had time for the hopeless, the potentially unproductive people who needed attention. Praise the Lord! *Somebody still cared!*

Twenty minutes finally dragged by, and I anxiously dialed the number to Dr. Schut's office. The receptionist on the other end already had my name and was expecting my call. She explained that Dr. Schut was out of town and that he was scheduled to return late Monday. (This was Thursday.) She gave me an appointment to see him on Tuesday. I thanked her and hung up.

I called Kitty back and cried as I told her how kind and helpful Dr. Koop had been and thanked her for her help. I told her that I planned to fly, so that David could stay at work and keep the boys and his life as normal as possible.

She inquired as to where I planned to stay. "At the hospital with Eric—I wouldn't dare leave him there alone!" I answered.

"Who will pick you up at the airport?" she continued.

"I guess I'll take a cab. I don't know anyone in Philadelphia," I said.

"Let me call you back after I talk with some friends. I think I could find someone to pick you up at the airport, anyway. At least you would get acquainted with some good Christian people and you wouldn't feel so alone," she insisted.

She didn't have to twist my arm. I consented. After all, it would seem strange not knowing anyone. Shortly—she called again, telling me a sweet Christian lady would meet me at the airport. Kitty was thinking of things my numb mind could not begin to comprehend, much less organize. I appreciated her so much at this moment in my life!

I sat down in my den with a sigh. Looking at the games on the book shelf that David Jr., Brian, and I used to play made me realize how much I missed doing things of that sort with my two little boys. It seemed it had been an eternity since I had felt like playing a game, or, for that matter, had been able to play a game, considering the constant care Eric had needed.

I began to dream of how wonderful it would be for Eric to improve enough so that I could once again be a decent mother to them—once again, I could be a decent wife.

When David would ventilate to me about his day at work, perhaps my mind would be clear enough to comprehend what he was saying, so that I could carry on a decent conversation. Once again, I could get some sleep, and my health would improve. I was looking forward to "reaching the mountain top." Eric and I had been plundering around in the "valley" long enough.

My thoughts were interrupted as I realized it was

time to feed Eric another half ounce of liquid. As I changed his diaper, I noticed he wasn't as responsive as he had been the last hour. I fed him his half ounce; his stomach rejected it.

I knew that I could not wait until Tuesday. I knew he must have intravenous fluids in order to survive. Perhaps if I were able to get him to Philadelphia, they could relieve enough pressure through his Rickham reservoir and give him intravenous fluids, enabling him to live until Dr. Schut returned.

I called Dr. Schut's office back and asked if his associate would talk with me. He returned my call in less than an hour. I told him that Eric's condition was such that I did not think he could survive until Tuesday without medical attention.

He assured me that he could take care of Eric until Dr. Schut returned. "Get him here as soon as you can. However, if you plan to fly, I would highly recommend that you have the neurosurgeon there tap the Rickham reservoir before you get on the plane. An inadequately pressurized aircraft could be very risky to a baby with increased intracranial pressure already," he said. I told him that I would, and thanked him.

I immediately phoned Dr. Johnson's office and told his receptionist to have him meet me in the emergency room. (He was already at the hospital, but not in surgery.) I hurriedly cancelled my plane reservations for Monday night and moved them up to that evening. My mother came over to help me pack, while I took Eric to see Dr. Johnson at the emergency room.

While we waited for Dr. Johnson, a lab technician came to draw blood from Eric. Soon Dr. Johnson arrived.

I began, "Dr. Johnson, Eric is very sick. I took him to the pediatrician this morning, and he could not find any infection. He's showing signs of increased intracranial pressure. Would you tap his Rickham reservoir to see if his pressure is at an intolerable level?"

He shook his head, negatively. He looked at Eric with his mouth slightly curled to the side and said, "He doesn't need his Rickham tapped."

I decided that I must be a little more explicit and honest now: "Dr. Johnson, I've decided to take him to Children's Hospital of Philadelphia. I talked with Dr. Koop by phone this afternoon. Do you know him?"

He shook his head. "His name doesn't sound familiar," he said.

"Well, the neurosurgeon in Philadelphia said that before I risked taking him on an inadequately pressurized aircraft, you should drain some fluid from his reservoir. I'm planning to fly with him this evening. Would you drain it for us?" (thinking that surely since another neurosurgeon had suggested it, he would oblige).

"Take him on the airplane; it won't hurt him." He continued, "What do you hope to accomplish up there?"

I looked at him for a moment. "Peace of mind, if nothing else," I answered.

He said, "I understand—well—take him on. The airplane trip won't hurt him."

I picked up Eric, and we left the hospital. Dr. Johnson never even waited to see his blood test results before he said "goodbye."

Upon returning home, I called the airline reservation agent and inquired about the pressurization of the aircraft. She asked why I was interested. When I explained the situation, she exclaimed, "Take that baby to Philadelphia some other way. There's no way we can promise adequate pressurization through an entire flight!"

After David and I discussed our predicament briefly, he decided the only safe alternative was for us to drive. I cancelled the plane reservations, and David made last minute preparations with his boss by phone to be off work the following day.

I made sure the children had eaten enough of the delicious supper my mother had prepared for them. I finished packing David a suitcase. He would have to stay somewhere overnight and catch up on the sleep he would lose from driving that night.

Our neighbor was a truck driver and offered to supply us with a map showing us the best route to take. We had never driven any farther north than Washington, D.C.; so this was a special blessing and comfort to us. He insisted we take his citizen band radio just in case Eric needed emergency medical attention during the trip.

I knew the hospital there would want the same type blood test that the lab technician had obtained at the emergency room. To save Eric an extra stick in his arm, I called the lab and wrote the results down as the clerk read them off to me.

Time flew by, and it was bedtime for David Jr. and Brian before we left. As I took time to tuck them in, I could tell they were worried. I tried to tell them how much I loved them, and I did not want to leave them; but it was necessary. "If you were sick, and the doctors here could not help you, I would take you anywhere—no matter how far—to get the best care for you."

They were tearful but seemed to understand why we had to go. I fought back my tears, as I walked into my room to get the suitcases.

I noticed Mother crying as she stood beside Eric's crib.

"Are you afraid he's going to die?" I asked.

"Well, the Lord hasn't answered my prayer," she said.

"What did you pray?"

"I prayed that He would be able to use the doctors here."

"Well, for some reason he isn't going to. Mother, there's no doubt in my mind that the Lord is directing us to Philadelphia. Now quit crying. Eric is not going to die! The Lord is going to heal him. I know He is!" I hurriedly threw some articles into the suitcase and closed it.

"I just can't bear to watch him suffer. He's the worst I've ever seen him!" Mother continued to weep as she spoke.

I wanted to put my arms around her and tell her that everything was going to be all right, and thank her for being my mother. She had stood by us through thick and thin.

Several times, when I had reached the point that I could no longer go on physically, she would come over and care for Eric while I got some rest. Now, I knew I could count on her to be dad and mom to my boys while we were done.

I wanted to tell her how much I loved her and appreciated her, but the lump in my throat was too big. The words wouldn't come. I didn't want her to see me cry. She would worry about us as we drove all night. Mothers are like that. No matter how old we get, we never get independent of mother's love and worry.

David's mother lived several miles away. He had called to tell her our plans. She wouldn't sleep much, either. She had always been there for us. She, too, would share the load of caring for our boys in our absence. The only concern I had regarding their care was that they weren't very good disciplinarians. They didn't have any trouble spanking us when we were growing up, but for some reason they "forgot how" when they became grandmothers.

Moments later, we said "goodbye" and began our long drive. I persuaded David to let me drive to Washington while he rested. I argued that I could never sleep riding, while he could. "Besides," I continued, "I know my way to Washington; and it's better for one of us to get some rest than for neither of us to sleep." He very reluctantly consented. I had not slept the night before.

The Lord miraculously gave me strength and alertness as I drove. Every hour I continued to give Eric fluid through a nasogastric tube as he lay on a pillow between us. He was past being irritable now, and he lay almost lifeless during the entire trip. I would rest my right hand on his back periodically to make sure I could feel him breathing.

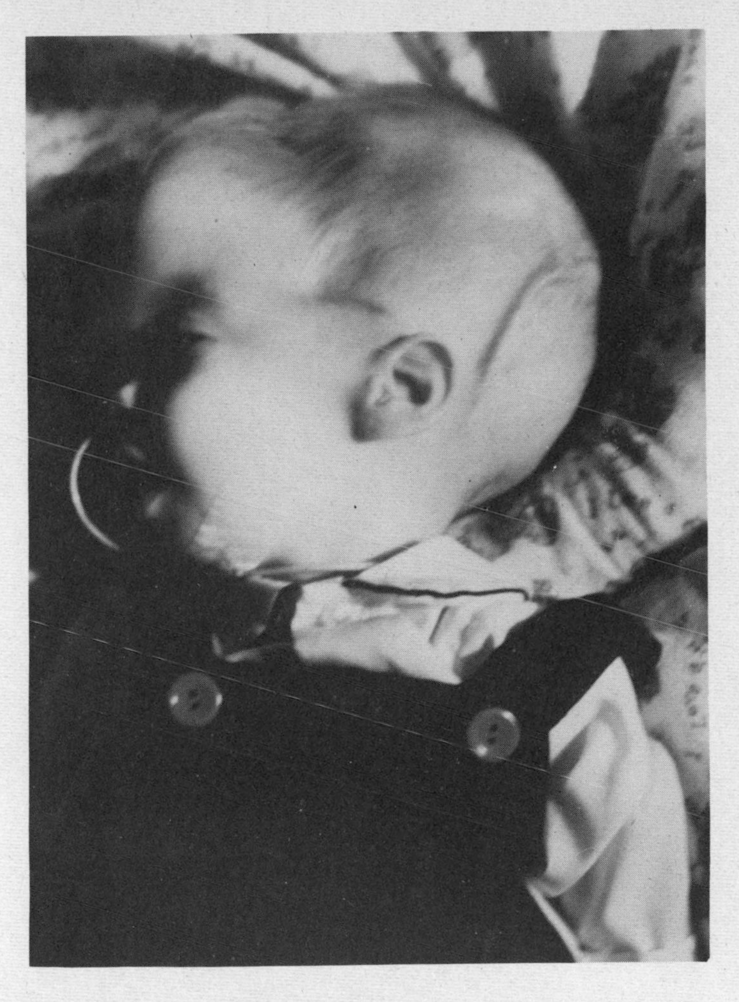

The tiny tube just beneath the skin on Eric's skull is his new double-barrel shunt.

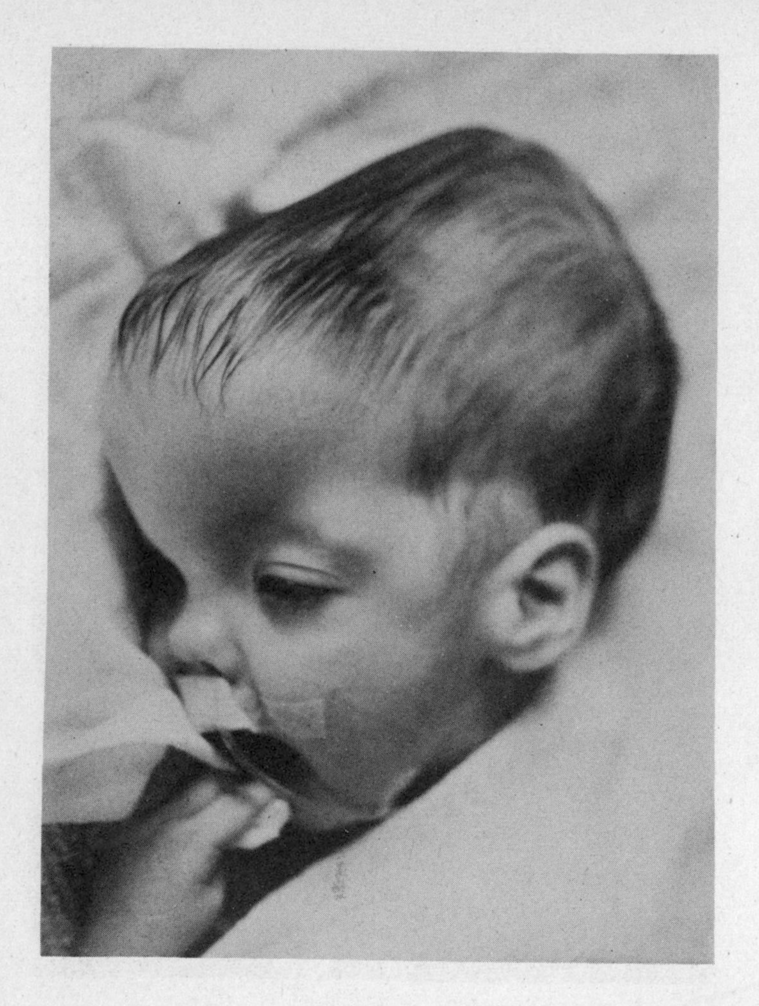

Eric became more alert and active after his hospitalization at Philadelphia.

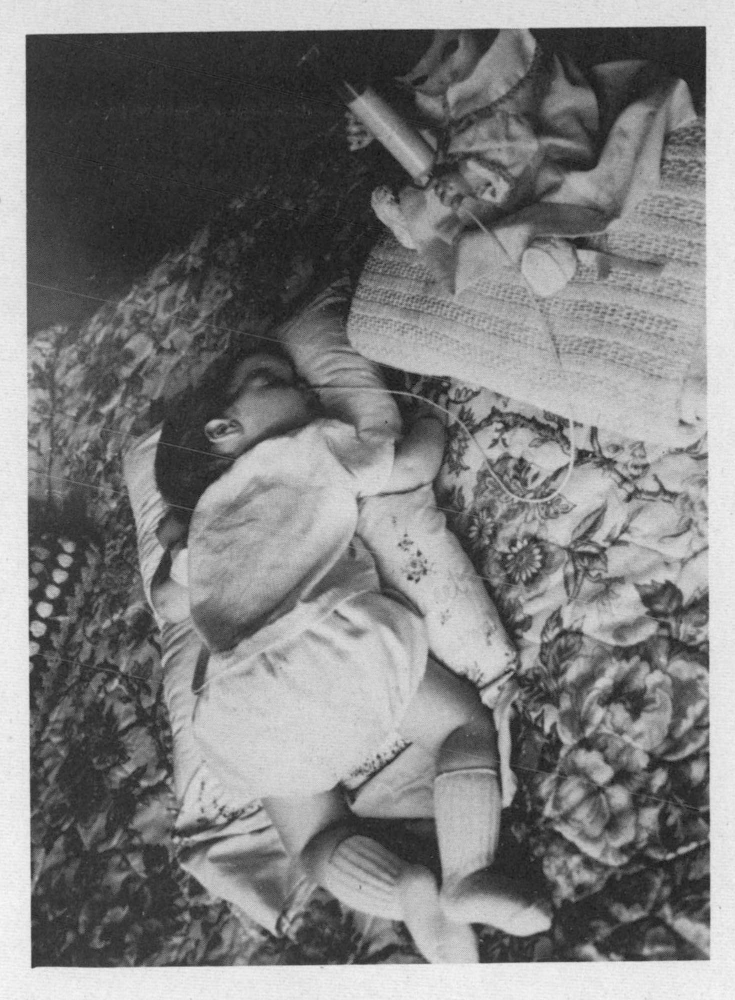

A doll from girlhood served as a handy nurse aid for tube feedings while I folded diapers nearby.

11

Daybreak

Light began to break across the Philadelphia horizon. As we drove through the early morning traffic, I couldn't help but wonder if this dawn had a special meaning for us. We stopped once to ask directions to Children's Hospital and found our way without difficulty. For newcomers, that within itself was something to praise the Lord for.

Upon our arrival Dr. Schut's associate saw Eric without delay. After looking at the brain scans we had brought, he took Eric into his arms. Needless to say, Eric did not put on his best performance! He lay without initiative, only fretting weakly when agitated.

"I can see now by looking at the scans why the doctors weren't very optimistic about Eric," he began. "The only reason that he is still living is because you're a nurse; and if he lives, it will only be because of the care you give him. This little fellow will probably never be independent of you. He may say a few words, but will most probably never walk. There's no way of predicting how long he may live." He paused.

"I understand why you feel this way; however, this baby showed good potential of being normal until he was three months old," I said.

"Well, we will run some tests on him this morning to help us determine how much brain function we may be dealing with," he continued; "however, I believe we still can help him with the fluid in his brain. We have had success with what we call a double-barrel shunt. With this procedure, all Eric's ventricles will be drained equally, perhaps causing an improvement where his vomiting is concerned. We will admit Eric and attempt to get him well hydrated with intravenous fluids, and I will tap the Rickham reservoir. This should keep him a little more comfortable while we wait for Dr. Schut to return."

As he spoke to his receptionist regarding the tests he wanted to be run on Eric, his words again ran through my mind: "I can see now by looking at the scans why the doctors weren't very optimistic about Eric . . . This little fellow will probably never be independent of you."

"Did we drive all night to hear this?" I thought to myself. He explained that a pediatrician would also be seeing Eric and told his receptionist to show us to the location where an EEG (a test showing the brain waves) would be done.

When we left his office, the Lord brought to my mind a very special verse in Psalm 112:7:

> "He shall not fear evil tidings; his heart is fixed, trusting in the Lord."

It was such a comfort as we walked down the corridors to the EEG lab.

As we were sitting waiting for them to call us, I looked at my exhausted, red-eyed husband, and asked, "Honey, what did you think of what the doctor said?"

"You want me to be honest?"

"Yes." I feared what was coming next. Was his faith getting weak?

"I'm so tired that I can't think." he answered.

What a relief! He was too tired to try to comprehend the doctor's prognosis. I told him that I felt Eric was still going to surprise everyone.

The technician ran the most thorough EEG that I've ever witnessed. I was impressed with his knowledge and ability. He didn't hesitate to answer all of my many questions.

Afterwards, we took our son to have a visual evoked response test (abbreviated VER, testing to see how fast his brain responded to a bright light, flashed repeatedly at different speeds at a certain distance from his face).

I figured he'd fail this test miserably, since the squirt would not open his eyes. The technician explained that it wasn't necessary for him to open his eyes. As the test was in progress, he asked, "How old did you say this baby was?"

"Ten-and-a-half months."

"He's doing as well as the babies we've tested at one year old!"

"Praise the Lord for one good piece of news!" I thought. Then replied, "That's good."

Eric was admitted to the fifth floor. Three other babies shared his room. I watched intently and was impressed with the excellent nursing care.

David found a room in a nearby hotel. He agreed to return later so that I could use the room to shower and change. I couldn't believe I was still awake after more than forty-eight hours. The Lord's strength was more than sufficient.

Later that evening, two pediatric resident doctors came to Eric's bedside. One spoke to the other, "Let's take him into the treatment room."

As they started to pick up Eric I questioned, "Wait, what are you going to do?"

"A spinal tap to rule out meningitis."

"I haven't signed anything giving you permission to do this!" I exclaimed.

"You don't have to sign for a spinal tap here."

"Well, we do back home; and whether or not I have to sign up here, I still want you to ask my permission before doing procedures such as this," I said firmly, so they could have no doubt as to my feelings.

"Well, the doctor has ordered it; and we're just doing what we've been told to do."

"What doctor?" I asked.

"The neurosurgeon," one resident answered.

"I don't mean to be offensive; but if the neurosurgeon wants a spinal tap done, then I would rather he did the procedure."

"Why? We do more spinal taps than the doctors."

"That may be true; however, I did not bring him here for the best medical students to experiment on. I brought him here for the best doctors to look after him."

They looked quite annoyed as they attempted to gain my confidence by making statements such as; "we do these all the time without any trouble," etc. I believe I was the first stubborn mother they had encountered.

I told the nurse to call the neurosurgeon so that I could speak with him by phone. I knew I must make my wishes known to him, so there would be no misunderstandings as to what I expected of Eric's care. She did as I asked.

I began, "Doctor, I know Eric is unique in several ways, and I don't mind residents learning from him; but if they learn, they'll do so by watching the attending physicians do the procedures.

"We didn't drive all night to have medical students look after our baby. At home, I had the very best looking after Eric, and I did not tolerate resident doctors getting practice on him. I was told the best would look after him here, and I won't settle for less!"

"What seems to be the problem at the present?" he asked quietly.

"There's a couple of pediatric residents who want to do a spinal tap. They said you ordered it."

"Yes, I feel we need one, and they do more spinal

taps than we attending physicians do."

"Well, I'd be ashamed to admit that! I'd still rather you would do it."

"I can, but I feel they can do just as good a job as I. Since they are already there, why don't you permit them to go ahead with it this time? I feel confident they won't have any problems."

"Okay," I agreed, "but they better not make any mistakes with him!"

As Eric was taken into the treatment room, I prayed, "Lord, I don't want to be ugly; please give me wisdom about this situation. I don't want them sticking Eric's spine over and over again. He's so sick and frail."

I knew a good, successful spinal tap should take no longer then ten minutes. I waited thirty minutes; Eric still had not been brought back to his bed. I was sure they were having trouble.

I went to the nurses' station and asked Eric's nurse to check and see if they had gotten in yet. (By that, I meant had the spinal needle been injected into the right location.) In a few seconds she returned, saying that they had not been successful with it as yet.

"Then, please go tell them to pull out, clean Eric up, and bring him back to his room. If the neurosurgeon still wants a spinal tap, he can do it when he has time!" I ordered rather dogmatically.

She did as I asked, and the resident doctor came out complaining he didn't have the right equipment. He explained, "This is why it has taken so long. I have called the senior resident to try the tap."

"I'm sorry; I don't want any residents doing the tap. Just bring Eric back to his room!" I commanded.

"Then, I'll have to call the neurosurgeon," he replied.

"Fine, just tell him Eric's mother stopped the procedure. He'll understand," I said.

Thus, I proceeded to make enemies on Eric's first night of hospitalization in Philadelphia. I did what I felt I had to do for his benefit, regardless who it offended.

****

Let me stop here and say that the parent can control who has direct contact with his sick child from lab technicians all the way to the doctors! I only permitted two specific lab technicians in my hospital back home to draw blood because of their gentleness and success in obtaining his blood. I quickly learned who was careless and who was proficient.

Request whom you want. If it doesn't work, then *demand* whom you want for specific procedures. All personnel should wear name tags. Look at them. Find out your preference. The patient is paying dearly for good care and should never settle for less!

I cannot praise enough the nursing care Eric received at Philadelphia. In fact, the same two residents that I interrupted doing Eric's spinal tap were very kind to me later. We developed a good rapport before Eric's discharge.

I would also like to emphasize that on occasion, a

patient or a patient's family will develop a better rapport with a resident doctor than with their own attending physician.

Many times attending physicians have so many patients that they depend heavily on resident doctors (supposedly under their guidance) to do many of their duties. Therefore, resident doctors have more contact with the patients, frequently giving more needed individualized care.

It is not the purpose of this book to put "thumbs down" on any one group or type of doctors. I thank the Lord for the resident doctor who was concerned enough to make the sonograms of me during my pregnancy.

Further realize that when you or your family member is hospitalized, the patient, or parent, has a right to know exactly what is planned for his care. When the situation is not immediately life-threatening a parent should not allow any medical person to come into a room and remove their child from that room to perform a medical procedure without a satisfactory explanation of *what* the procedure is and *why* it needs to be done!

If the parent is still unsure of the explanation or need for the procedure; or is perhaps uncomfortable with the person who is to perform it, he can refuse to have the procedure performed until these specifications meet his approval.

Many times when patients are abnormal or terminally ill, they become human "guinea pigs" for students in the medical profession. I resent this and feel strongly that family members should be *cautious* and *explicit* regarding the care these patients receive.

These individuals usually do require more tests; therefore, the family should feel confident that the person who obtains the test will do so with the least amount of difficulty and discomfort to their loved one.

Read thoroughly any consent forms you sign. Make sure of your preference as to which doctor will perform the operation or procedure. The doctor's name should be on the permit.

When a parent remains with a child throughout an entire hospitalization, there's no need to sign a "blanket" consent form for "anything that may need to be done." The parent will be there to supervise the care and give permission as the child's individual needs arise.

When possible (and I would make every effort to make it feasible) a parent should stay with a hospitalized child aged seven and younger. It not only gives the child a needed sense of security and comfort, but the parent can do much of the time-consuming care, i.e., bathing, giving bedpans, and administering food and drink. Although nurses enjoy doing this care, the nationwide shortage of nurses is rapidly causing this personalized care to suffer.

For instance, I would prefer giving a child juice rather than a shot. Many times when I had three patients to inject, a child wanted juice (always immediately). A willing, available mother is such a blessing in these cases.

I have been on both sides of the fence now, both giving medical care and receiving it for myself and my child. I feel this advice, if used discreetly and kindly, will be profitable to patient care. If a patient is not receiving satisfactory care and attention, it is his right to obtain his records and seek help elsewhere.

****

The next morning the surgeon came to do Eric's spinal tap. He even offered to let me watch. We joked back and forth a little, then I declined his invitation.

When he brought Eric back to his room, I asked, "Have you seen any of Eric's function studies yet?"

He smiled slightly and said, "The VER was good. Maybe you're right about his potential." He had not been able to obtain the EEG results.

Later that afternoon, David kissed Eric and me goodbye and left to return home. I missed him, but the Lord's presence was so real. The nurses made me feel right at home.

Monday afternoon, Dr. Schut came in to visit. He told me that Eric's surgery was scheduled for one o'clock the following day. He would be putting in a double-barrel shunt, hoping to equalize the pressure and draining of fluid in his head. "Come to my office, and talk with my any time you like," he added cordially.

He had asked me to find the neurosurgeons' notes from the records I had brought with me; he said that he would pick them up later.

If anyone had told him what a particularly uncooperative mother I had been, he never let on.

Shortly, I found the neurosurgeons' notes, and took them down to his office.

When I handed him the notes, he took a picture and showed me the parts of Eric's brain that were not normal. He made his condition very clear. He did not give a poor prognosis. He still contented that Eric had a "lot of good brain to work with."

"Well, Dr. Schut, I've prayed the Lord would lead me to a doctor who could help Eric; and I have no doubt He's led me to you. I know you have a lot of parents coming to this hospital hoping for miracles. I'm not hoping for one; neither am I expecting you to perform one. The Lord has already promised me that He was going to heal Eric (Psalm 138:8).

"Now, you say that you will be able to help his fluid problem. I feel the Lord led us here for that. Whatever else needs to be made normal about his brain, the Lord is able to do. There's nothing impossible with Him," I smiled confidently.

"You're right," he agreed.

I was surprised he didn't look at me as if I were weird.

He continued, "If all goes well then, we'll do his shunt tomorrow."

I thanked him for his time and left feeling nice inside that my little son had someone who cared and realized God still specializes in the impossible.

Shortly after returning to my room, I was visited by a nurse whom I used to work with back home. It was so comforting to see a familiar face. "What caused you to come up here?" she asked. When I told her that I had talked to Dr. Koop by phone, she said with emphasis; "*You* talked to *Dr. Koop?*"

"Sure, what's wrong with that?"

"Do you know who Dr. Koop is?!"

"He's the nicest doctor I've ever spoken to on the phone," I answered. "That's good enough for me."

"Jennifer, Dr. Koop has just been made *Surgeon General of the United States*! It's been all over the newspaper! Where have you been?"

I laughed, "Taking care of this baby, reading my Bible, and writing my book—I haven't had time to read newspapers."

After she left, I wept once again, thinking about how good the Lord had been; and I didn't even know it at the time. There I was back home, batting my head against the wall—looking for a doctor—begging well-respected physicians to just look at him—making desperate, fruitless efforts—becoming discouraged to the point of finally saying, "Lord, if you don't guide us, we're doomed!" (Psalm 119:126).

He looked down and said, "Poor Jennifer, I was wondering when she would give up and trust Me completely."

The Lord knew the Surgeon General of the United States personally. I did not. He knew how to put me through the right channels to get to him. There was the concerned pediatrician He used and a godly missionary with a sweet little boy who had a birth defect; and I wouldn't be surprised if the Lord didn't put Dr. Koop exactly where I could get in touch with him when I needed him most. He very easily could have been out to lunch or out of the country.

How very real the verses are now:

> "I called upon the Lord in distress; the Lord answered me, and set me in a large place. The Lord is on my side; I will not fear: . . . The Lord taketh my part with them that help me . . . It is better to trust in the Lord than to put confidence in man.
>
> Psalm 118:5-8

Just before Eric's surgery, the anesthesiologist came to talk with me. It seemed all the children on the floor were catching a "bug" of some sort. Eric couldn't be left out and decided he would pick up a stuffy nose and fever. The anesthesiologist explained that the surgery took priority above the upper respiratory infection. "However," he continued, "there's an increased risk of him getting into respiratory distress and ending up in ICU on a ventilator. You being a nurse should understand the potential problem."

I nodded. I was "a nurse," yes; but I was all "mother" now, and didn't particularly want to hear about the "potential problems." But I knew he was obligated to tell me.

After he left, I asked the Lord to keep Eric from problems and to please permit him to return to his room after surgery. The nurse came in to prepare him, and I knew it wouldn't be long before they came to get him.

He still wasn't very responsive. I hovered close to his little ear and sang softly. Then I told him, "Jesus is going to make you better."

It seemed that just for a moment the devil crept

up and whispered in my ear, "Are you sure Jesus is going to make him better? Here you are in this strange place all by yourself. How are you going to feel if you have to fly back with Eric in a casket instead of in your arms?"

I said silently, firmly, "Get thee behind me, Satan. I'm not alone; and I'll be traveling back with Eric in my arms, so be on your way!"

The operating room personnel permitted me to go with Eric into a holding area. Eric and I were to wait there until the anesthesiologist came for him. His chart was lying on the end of the stretcher. I figured that reading it would be an interesting way to pass the time; besides, I was especially interested to see if his EEG report was there.

As I picked it up, a clerk quickly grabbed it and said, "I need to look at this for a moment."

I chuckled to myself as I watched her call a nurse from the operating room nurses' station. She whispered a few words and then the nurse said aloud, "You have to give it back to her. It's her right."

The clerk brought it back and handed it to me. I proceeded to read it. I was as impressed with the nurses' efficiency in charting as I was the care they gave.

I hurried for fear they would come before I skimmed over everything. I found the EEG report. It said that Eric's EEG was *"within normal limits for his age."*

I was thrilled!

How dare the devil try to tell me that I was all alone! "I'd like to kick him in the teeth!" I thought.

We waited only a short time before the anesthesiologist came.

The surgery was successful, and he was brought back to his room. Praise the Lord! A few hours later, one of the pediatric residents came in and looked at Eric. I had put his favorite little yellow bear in his crib. He was lying in a position where he could look at it.

"Mrs. Vanderford!" the resident said excitedly, looking at him a second time, "He's smiling! Did you know he's smiling?"

I laughed, "Yes, I know. He can do more than smile, but I'm having a hard time making anyone believe that he has potential."

"I'm beginning to think you may be right!"

It was nice to see Eric smile again. It had been almost two months since I had seen it.

He was discharged from the hospital four days later. And began to improve by leaps and bounds. He gained strength as he put on three pounds the first three weeks we were home. The vomiting stopped. His muscle tone improved. He began to laugh and coo when we gave him attention. The shape of his head improved. I could not praise the Lord enough!

At six o'clock on the morning of March 29, 1981, I sat down beside Eric's crib and watched as he slept peacefully on his first birthday. Tears fell down my cheeks once again as I sang "Happy Birthday" to him. I also sang the second verse which goes:

Happy birthday to you
Only one will not do

Born again means salvation
Then you will have two.
(*Action Songs for Children*, Volume I)

I picked up a pencil lying nearby and wrote:

Today's your special day, dear one,
Granted sweetly by God's dear Son.
Just sang the birthday song to you
And told you that you must have two.
The second one, of course, will be
When you receive the One on Calvary.
Then He'll show you the path to take,
Reveal the purpose for which you were
made.
Just follow Him, Eric, and you will be
great.
The trials and miracles have been no
mistake.
You've been protected and cared for by
the Unseen Hand,
Singled out as a vessel for a special plan.
Can't wait to see what the Lord's going
to do
To manifest His works through you!

Love,
Mother

Epilogue

I can honestly say if Eric should die today, he already has been more than a blessing sent from above. This experience has taught me to be totally dependent on the Lord Jesus, to rest completely in His promises, and to actually thrive from day to day on His Word. I can say as the Psalmist:

> "Before I was afflicted I went astray: but now have I kept thy word . . . It is good for me that I have been afflicted; that I might learn thy statutes. The law of thy mouth is better unto me than thousands of gold and silver . . . Therefore I love thy commandments above gold; yea, above fine gold."
>
> Psalm 119:67, 71-72, 127

God has used Eric's condition to mold me into a vessel more fit for His use.

> "For thou, O God, hast proved us; thou hast tried us, as silver is tried."
>
> Psalm 66:10.

Are the trials for Eric over? I do not know, but—

> "He knoweth the way that I take: when he hath tried me, I shall come forth as gold."
>
> Job 23:10

—of Eric—

Not chastisement, but a blessing;
Not a burden, but a joy;
If you see us, don't glance with pity;
We're quite pleased with our little boy!

—of his future—

> "For our heart shall rejoice in him, because we have trusted in his holy name."
>
> Psalm 33:21

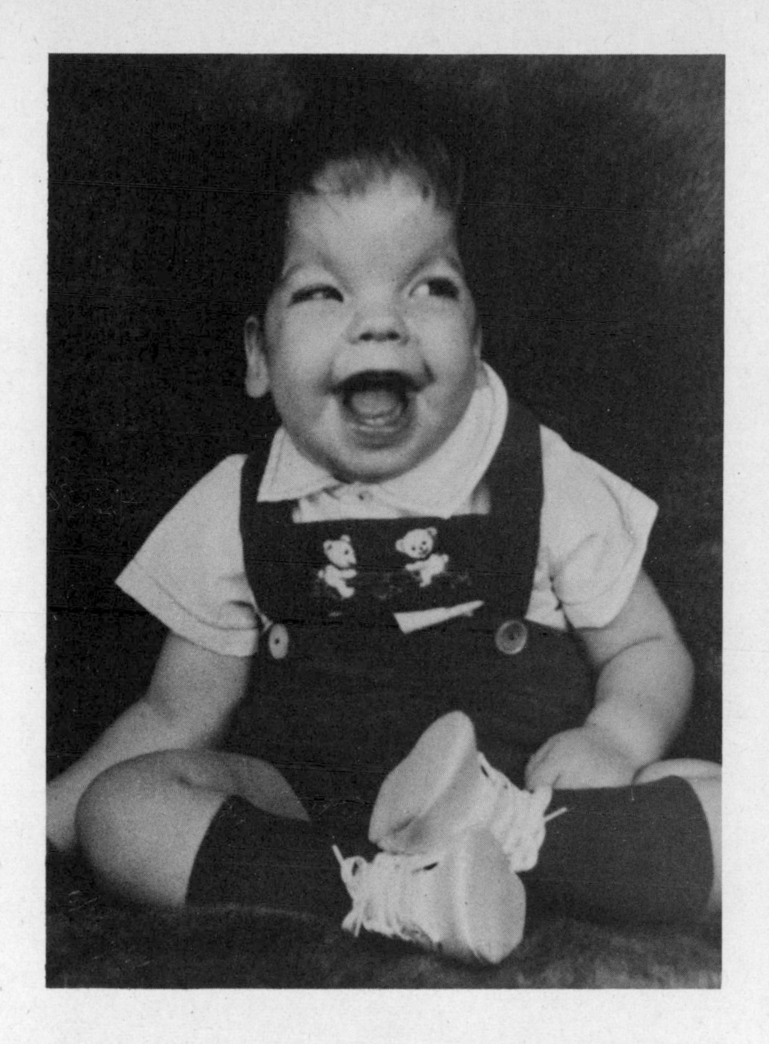

Eric, Christmas 1981, "Now unto him that is able to do exceedingly abundantly above all that we ask or think . . ."

Ephesians 3:20